The Breakaway

The Breakaway

A Parent's Guide to Transitioning the
Autistic and Twice Exceptional Adolescent
Into Young Adulthood

The Breakaway

ISBN: 9798656424431 (Paperback)

Library of Congress Control Number: 2021904864

Any references to historical events, real people, or real places are used fictitiously. Names, characters, and places are products of the author's imagination.

Cover art and design by Jeff Ignaszewski
Edited by Frank Mugavero

Published in the United States of America

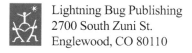 Lightning Bug Publishing
2700 South Zuni St.
Englewood, CO 80110

Acknowledgments

Writing a book has proven to be harder and more rewarding than I could have ever imagined. And while many hours were spent alone at a computer, this book's completion would not be possible without the inspiration, support, and encouragement of others.

I have to start by thanking my wife Laura and son Caleb. From the reading of early drafts, to your consistent encouragement, endless patience, and for not letting me quit, you both are the motivation I needed to keep moving forward. Thank you!

A special thanks to my editor Frank Mugavero. Your friendship, feedback, patience, and truly extraordinary editing skills have been invaluable to the completion of this project. I am forever grateful.

To Jeff Iggy for lending your time and artistic vision, and to Andy for being so willing to share your talents. Thank you both.

Finally, I want to thank the many parents and Breakaways that have inspired this project. It is my great honor to have worked with you all.

The Breakaway

Table of Contents

The Breakaway

Introduction

The Breakaway

If you are a parent or family member charged with supporting a teenager who is on the Autism Spectrum or identified as Twice Exceptional, there is one thing I already know about you...

Your time is very, very valuable.

So I am not going to waste your time with complicated theory or soothing platitudes. I'll just tell you who I am and why this book can help you.

My name is Tom Welch. I am a child and family psychologist with over 25 years of experience working with neurodiverse young people and their families. I specialize in work with those on the autism spectrum, and those who have been identified as Twice Exceptional (2e). And it is that quarter-century of experience, the hundreds of children and parents I have counseled over the years, which has informed and road-tested all the strategies I offer in this book.

Even more importantly, I am an educator.

As the owner and administrator of the Humanex Academy in Englewood, Colorado, I have the privilege of working hands-on every single day with teenagers struggling to fully understand and manage their learning differences, giving me a very practical understanding of what helps them and what doesn't.

In my capacity there, the two questions I am most often asked are *"What is it about your school that works so well?"* and *"Why is it called Humanex?"* The answer to both questions is really the same, and they both very much relate to the principles behind this book. The name refers to our philosophy of recognizing the unique history and personality of every student we teach, and the importance of always making room for the human experience in education (thus Human-Ex). That standard, and the curriculum it inspires, is what I believe makes our approach so effective.

Each of our students have their own specific set of goals and stumbling blocks – a stubborn individuality that resists a One-Size-Fits-All solution. The Humanex approach is about recognizing and appreciating those differences. We challenge them to look beyond their clinical diagnosis to the bigger picture of who they are and who they can be; to take pride in their personal identity and avoid the trap of comparing their progress with others.

We encourage boldness and optimism. After all, one cannot discover one's potential if everything is approached from a defensive position. Simple deficit remediation, or focusing on "not doing things wrong," is unhelpful for the neurodiverse student. It may feel better to avoid any chance of rejection or failure, but it leads only to self-fulfilling disappointment and diminishing returns.

3

Success both during and after high school requires the development of initiative, motivation, determination, and resilience. The formation of these skills will not develop within a vacuum. Instead, they must be taught to experiment, make mistakes, experience disappointment, AND to rebound within the real-world. This is also essential to the formation of a more mature sense of self that is distinct from others and critical for a successful push toward independence.

It is why I call my students approaching graduation *"The Breakaways"*.

Let's face it, graduating high school and making one's way into adulthood is the biggest and most daunting life transition many of us will ever face. There is discomfort, uncertainty and fear. Every step we take seems fraught with repercussions that could last the rest of our lives. We desperately want to "get it right". Often we are so afraid of making a mistake we become paralyzed with indecision. The pressure, the responsibility – it's all too much too soon.

Now imagine facing this scary time with the added baggage of an autism diagnosis or learning disability, making it exponentially more difficult and complicated.

Unlike their neurotypical peers, who likely faced equal measures of achievement and failure as they grew up, those with any level of neurodiversity have been dealt a disproportionate amount of setbacks and few victories to provide balance. No matter what their strengths, being 2e, their deficits are always what get the spotlight. When all the focus is on a person's limitations, desires get deferred, self-discovery is put on a shelf, and "The Future" is discussed with dread, rather than hope and promise.

Add the fact this population matures at a slower pace, often falling into a confusing limbo between chronological and experiential age, and it quickly becomes clear how crucial it is they begin to step out on their own, to exercise some autonomy.

Hence the term "Breakaway".

If that word still feels a little scary to you, triggers concern and anxiety, then congratulations: You're a good parent and you have done your job well.

Nevertheless, if their growth and development is to continue, your Breakaway needs to confront fresh challenges on his or her own. Which means your role has changed. ***Your job now is to be more like a coach.*** Not pushing or pulling them, but guiding them through this gauntlet, cheering them from the sidelines, challenging them when necessary, while making sure they don't get stuck, discouraged, or roam too far off track. Success is no longer defined simply by good grades or passing a class, but rather by your Breakaway falling down and getting back up again.

As they navigate the obstacles that arise from their disabilities, the goal of the coach is to facilitate this messy process – the making of mistakes, even occasionally learning "the hard way" – without allowing *your own fears* to obstruct the Breakaway's true path and forward momentum.

It will be incredibly stressful, at times even overwhelming.

That is normal. In fact, that is the goal.

Yes, learning to function with independence will require lots of practice and advance preparation. However, only real-world experience can complete the process. This is where your Breakaway will encounter the unexpected, test their skills at full speed; where previous lessons that were once abstract finally take hold and prove useful; and where undiscovered gaps in skill development are identified and resolved.

Despite the many setbacks that will occur, it is ultimately this difficult process of learning to navigate the challenges of exploration and discovery, that will give them a whole new level of confidence. The process is the goal, the goal is the process. If you go in understanding that every "crisis" bears the gift of growth, then you won't fall into panic mode – you will be able to stay calm and project calm, teaching them to react the same.

Being able to allay the fears of my students and their families, to help them through such a critical time, has been my most satisfying role as a psychologist.

While there are many books on the market about this population, I have never been able to find one that dealt specifically with this narrow but tricky juncture of late adolescence/ early adulthood and all the complicated choices it presents. It seemed to me parents needed something along the lines of a guidebook they could use with some flexibility on a day-by-day basis. One that doesn't cling to one standardized rote style of therapy/support, but offers many different strategies based on real individual case histories, as I do within these pages. With this approach I want to help you develop a plan and strategy that makes the most sense for you and your Breakaway. I will not be presenting a One-Size-Fits-All approach for you to implement. That would simply be a waste of everyone's time.

In the following chapters, we will talk about evaluating your Breakaway's current status and their *Readiness For Change*, the importance of setting the correct *Expectations* and giving good *Feedback*, dealing with the awkwardness of *Identity Development*, creating a culture of *Accountability*, allowing for the *Resilience* factor, projecting *Commitment*, as well your own learning curve as a parent and *Human Experience*.

At the end of each chapter, I am going to ask you a few questions so you can apply the issues raised to your own situation. This is where the development of your own unique plan and strategy begins. It goes without saying there are no right or wrong answers, and these are just offered so you might gain new insights into your young person and their development. I would strongly recommend, however, you consider writing your answers down at the end of each chapter, or in a notebook/journal all your own. This will enable you to record and return to your observations, thoughts and feelings at each stage of the process, and get the clarity that one often finds in working out a problem on paper. Additionally, I suggest that you recruit others on your support team to join you in this process. The resulting support and collaboration will be invaluable.

At the very back of the book, I have included a sample of just such a journal by one of my student's parents, with an expanded case study, and you can flip to the back and refer to it whenever you want. But please feel free to ignore it as well and make your journal in whatever form works for you.

In closing, I would also like you to know that I too am a parent. My experience as a father has shaped much of the work I do and the perspective I take in this book.

And though my son, Caleb, is only 8 as I write this, I watch in awe as his special one-in-a-billion personhood takes shape before me and my wife's eyes with each new day.

When I watch him play, I am reminded of what naturalist John Muir once said: "The power of imagination makes us infinite." To become anything, we first need to imagine it. To see it in our mind. To believe. This is what Breakaways need most and what we must steer them towards…the power to imagine a full life. It may demand more work and time, but the challenges posed by an Autism or 2e diagnosis should not restrict or place any chains on their dreams.

This transition, however scary, is the start of realizing those dreams.

Onward!

T.W.

Notes

The Breakaway

Readiness For Change

*The curious paradox is that when
I accept myself just as I am,
then I can change.*

Carl Rogers

Given you are reading this book, it is safe to assume you are all too aware of the hurdles that lie ahead for your Breakaway after graduation and the need to create a well-drawn strategy moving forward. You are ready, anxious even, to take those next steps.

Unfortunately, your developing (or "aspiring" at this point) young adult may not be. They may not share your sense of urgency.

In fact, in certain ways, they may remain oblivious that their life needs any change or advance at all. And this can be extremely frustrating. Especially when you have devoted enormous resources to this transition and their achievements to date. Many parents respond to this paralysis and evasion with a blunt force approach – a demand for instant maturity on a tight time-table and at all costs. The neurodiverse teen naturally sees this as confrontational, not supportive, and everything comes to a standstill as a power struggle ensues.

To avoid this unproductive impasse, you must take into account their current strug-gle, any fear or indecision, and learn to push in a manner that does not alienate, but rather res-onates with their needs. Remember, a lack of forward movement or even resistance to change is not a personal flaw, and never as simple as "laziness" or apathy. It is a normal reaction for someone with their limited experience. The Breakaway who doesn't struggle to step outside their familiar world is the exception to the rule – change almost never comes without a fight.

This process is about helping them move beyond their easy generalized dreams of independence to grasp the hard work and specific goals required to get there.

So, how do you do that?

In this chapter I am going to tell you how to best evaluate their current emotional state and assess how ready they are for the enormous changes in store; how to recognize what ***Stage Of Change*** they currently occupy, so you can modify your approach appropriately.

But, before we start, I want to stress a few basic principles…

First, you need to listen.

This may seem like simplistic, even patronizing advice – but it is the first rule of any working partnership, the new dynamic you are hoping to foster with your Breakaway. And, sad to say, often the first casualty in a family's mad dash toward High School graduation.

Before doing anything else, take time to really observe and listen.

Remember, you are starting over. You are at square one again, and though it is scary for both of you, it is also a gift. It is an opportunity to communicate more openly, to show respect for their new status, and to find out who they are right now, in this moment.

You need to listen not only to what your Breakaway is saying, but to the feelings and meaning behind the stories and frustrations they share.

While you may have been on this journey through childhood and adolescence with them, as the one on the frontline, their experience is still very different than yours – and, obviously, what is most important. Demonstrating you recognize that essential truth is a powerful way to build the connection needed for the journey ahead.

This involves reflecting back to your young adult the feelings they share that seem most impactful and dominant in their present state, whether it is anxiety, anger, impatience, self-doubt, hope, or determination. It cannot just be a rote parroting of what you hear though. It should be an interpretation that shows a genuine understanding or desire to understand. It does not have to be complicated either. *"It's frustrating to feel like you have to work harder than others"*, *"This is a scary transition"*, or *"It's exciting to imagine living on your own"*, are all great jumping-off points for more in-depth conversations.

You do not need to feel the pressure to be exceptionally insightful. Or even "right" all the time. Rather, it is the simple acknowledgment of their experience that is most significant. It is even okay to question your perceptions and ask for clarification if you are unsure. For example, *"As I listen to what you are saying, it sounds like you are feeling unsure about your ability to adjust to living away from home. Am I understanding you correctly?"*

Besides giving you a real-time assessment of their wants and their worries, it has the added benefit of allowing them to teach you.

In my experience, almost all young neurodiverse adults feel that people do not take them seriously, or grasp what they are trying to say or do. They feel disrespected and misunderstood. These feelings result from their already long history of struggle. Because of their social awkwardness, many peers, or even teachers and other adults, have written them off almost without a thought; responding in negative ways ranging from casual dismissal to total humiliation. Over time, these interactions accumulate and leave behind scar tissue.

Imagine just a small sampling of the cuts and bruises they have sustained:

How could you not like more than pasta to eat?
You can't possibly think YOU can do that?
You're odd.
I don't want to be your friend.
Do it better, faster, different, again...etc.

You can't possibly think YOU can do that?
This class is not for you.
You complicate things when you're around.
What are we even going to do with you?
You dress funny.

Sound familiar?

You may think they have forgotten all these comments and the pain associated with them, but... Always being ridiculed, called out as weird, having others repeatedly change topics of conversation away from one's area of interest, having one's opinion minimized or discounted, or simply being continuously corrected, is tough. The result is an increased sense of isolation and a poorly developed sense of their own instincts and abilities.

A loss of voice, you might say.

In response, many turn inward and remain dependent, while others try frantically to overcompensate and push away from anything that makes them feel like the "disabled" person they no longer want to be. However your Breakaway is responding, it is important to realize that many of the behaviors you observe during this transition are rooted in the past. That background is something you must work to understand and overcome. In the hurry to reach and check off the next stage of development, parents too often fall into the habit of just discounting their child's complaints and protestations. It is easy to do and is generally motivated by the best of intentions; but if your approach to the challenges ahead recalls negative memories for them, they are not going to respond well or work with you.

So, slow down. Take time to engage them on a different level than you have before. Do not make any assumptions. Do not dictate. Learn to respond to what you are hearing, not to what you want to hear or what you "know" needs to happen next.

The goal at this early stage is their acceptance that they cannot tackle certain challenges alone or with their existing skill set. They must demonstrate a willingness to look honestly at their strengths and weaknesses. To do this, they will need to feel you are a non-threatening resource on which to call upon, that they won't be judged or rushed, just assisted. And to feel that, they must feel they have been heard and understood.

While much of the early agenda will be shaped by you, it is very important the young adult realizes this is about a *collaboration*, not their compliance!

A relationship based in compliance may find immediate success when the authority figure is present, but the effects do not last long in their absence. Since your absence, or at least reduced involvement, in the daily life of your child is actually the ultimate goal here, this only leaves an approach of supportive collaboration.

It begins with asking for their active participation from the start, inviting them into the decision-making process in a way that confirms their identity as a Young Adult.

This is called *The Buy-In* and no success exists without it!

It is the most crucial component in forming a game plan the Breakaway will not only accept, but be invested in and excited about accomplishing.

Remember, you are a coach now.

What makes a great coach? It is someone who gets the best performance out of their "athlete" by, firstly, believing in them, secondly, inspiring them to keep expanding their abilities, and thirdly, encouraging them to follow the healthy habits that will make that possible. And they have to do all of this without being too dominant or negative, inhibiting the "athlete".

Learning how to influence and guide in a manner that is well-received, and subtly produces continuous improvement, is the sly craft and dark art of coaching.

Ensuring your young adult is completely on board, and excited enough to self-motivate and meet you halfway as partner, will require a great deal of that sly craft.

How high should I set the bar? How do I provide helpful feedback? When should I intervene (hint: rarely) and when must I resist that impulse (hint: often)? How do I push my Breakaway at the right pace? Not too fast, which may cause discouragement, but not too slow either, causing them to become bored, complacent, unmotivated. This is your new calculus. A great coach doesn't accept excuses, but always provides an environment of emotional security, a safe space for trial-and-error experimentation. They stay engaged but flexible, allowing for occasional lapses, adjusting their own unrealistic expectations when necessary.

Let go of the notion progress will conform to any specific time-table.

The traditional agenda for parenting a neurotypical young adult through this time by identifying a school, training program, job or vocational position of interest, followed by the application process, acceptance, enrollment, etc, while setting higher standards for personal responsibility, all of that applies to neurodiverse kids as well, just not on the same schedule. They will still need high levels of support beyond that of their same age peers. You must come to accept this reality and not let get in your way of providing appropriate levels of encouragement and coaching. A focus on momentum not milestones is key here. This may be the very first time these Breakaways have taken ownership of the daily decisions in their life, and they are being asked to do it in the least-structured atmosphere they have ever known. They are easily overwhelmed by an unfamiliar environment and new routines. Their recovery time is longer. For all these reasons, they require an approach that does not expect too much too soon, facilitates growth by building one success carefully upon another.

Just as their developmental trajectory was different from their peers at earlier ages, their evolution into adulthood will be on their own timeline.

And finally…

Expect to be challenged.

14

Throughout this whole process, even when things are going extremely well, your Breakaway will sometimes fight you for no reason, object and resist.

It is a projection of their own insecurity. They will test you and try to "push your buttons," in an effort to elicit an old reward or compel you to reflexively jump in and take over for them. Don't take the bait. Take it in stride and keep to your new working partnership. This new observational – *not passive!* – role requires patience and a restraint which might well feel counterintuitive at times. But, eventually, you will notice the less you intervene, the more positive change will occur spontaneously, on its own merit.

As I said, it is important to acknowledge and not minimize their feelings, but try not to "join the crisis", which is very easy to do. Instead, just assert your confidence in them and that they will be able to make the right decision, handle whatever comes their way.

Again, effective coaching comes down to influence, not control.

Maintaining a strong working relationship even when the inevitable conflict arises; promoting growth, not power struggles.

You're there to help them maintain forward momentum.

Okay, let's get started.

So, how can you know where your young adult currently stands in the Process?

That's where the **Stages of Change** model developed by psychologists James Prochaska and Carlo DiClemente comes in. It provides a solid framework with which to gauge their readiness. In most situations, a change in behavior occurs gradually, beginning from a place where individuals are uninterested, unaware or unwilling to make change (***Pre-Contemplation***). Then opening up, allowing a consideration for change (***Contemplation***), and then to a more committed place where preparations for change can be made (***Preparation***). Eventually, motivated, determined action is taken (***Action***). And finally, over time, attempts to maintain the new behavior are made (***Maintenance***).

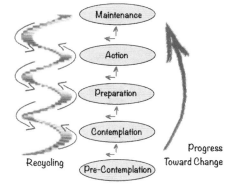

Recycling or Back-Sliding is an inevitability in this process, with the Breakaway cycling through these stages again and again until mastery has been achieved.

For our purposes, if we follow this structure, it gives us an effective guide for how and when parents should provide assistance, where to push, and when to step away.

Testing the Waters

Breakaways, just like most of their peers, expend a great deal of energy presenting an image to the world, a level of bravado or confidence seldom backed up by ability. They are "sure" they have things under control, and are reticent to accept feedback or the evaluation of others. For many it is a matter of pride. If siblings or people they know have not needed certain help, there is no way they are going to ask for or accept it.

This is why initiating the first conversation about their future is a delicate matter, and where a knowledge of the individual Stages of Change comes into play.

Using a measured approach, parents can begin with a relaxed "after hours" talk about the challenges ahead, decisions that must be made, etc. A testing of the waters. ***This is not the time to try to convince your Breakaway what to do*** – instead, use these initial discussions as a valuable opportunity for you to assess what stage they're at in the change process.

If these conversations show a lack of understanding of what is ahead, if you find yourself pushing, if you are exerting all the effort, or if they express complete disinterest, your young adult is in Stage One (Pre-contemplation). Stage Two responses (Contemplation) are more likely to acknowledge the challenge ahead and will have a broad sense of what they would like to become, but will lack a sense of the details. In response to your suggestions and encouragement you are likely to hear, "yes, but" statements, indicating they are not ready to consider next steps. This type of response largely defines stage two. Aware that change might be needed, while simultaneously, clinging to the familiar. An individual in Stage Three (Preparation), will more actively engage you in conversations about preparations to be made, and will have a building sense of determination for what they will face. They however are not yet fully on board and committed to taking action. They are still very reticent. A Stage Four (Action) individual is fully committed, has a strategy for moving forward, and is ready to take action. They will be very involved in goal-setting and will respond well to expectations for achievement. Stage Five (Maintenance) conversations will involve the sustaining of existing and well-established behaviors. While it is unlikely the majority of their skills will adapt smoothly, without complication, there will be some that will transfer well to life away from the structure of home and family. However, expect occasional lapses.

Let's go into this a little deeper, take it stage by stage.

Pre-Contemplation - Stage 1

Your goal here in this first stage is simply to engage them with empathy and thought-provoking questions. For example, ***"How are you going to live independently if...?"***, ***"What are the good things about living with us, being dependent on our support?"***, ***"What*** *are the bad things?", "I know you would like to be more independent than you are"* or, *"Where do you want to be in five years? Why? How do you think that would that feel?"* It is important to maintain a positive and warm tone while posing these challenging questions. Their purpose is to increasingly highlight the need for change. **Your goal is NOT to create change at this point.** Instead, you are working to build insight and awareness. It is through the greater levels of awareness developed at this stage that first steps are initiated.

PARENTING STAGE ONE

Developmental Goal:
The goal for this stage is for the developing young adult to think about the possibility of change.

Strategies:
- Validate their lack of readiness and encourage evaluation of current behavior. Clarify that the decision is theirs to make, and assist with the identification of obstacles and behavioral observations.
- Explain and personalize the pros and cons of choosing to take on the challenge of change, and of not taking on this challenge.
- Encourage conversations about greater independence and not action. This knowledge will be put to good use when current behaviors are compared to those needed for greater independence.
- Assist with the identification of obstacles, and skills/behaviors needed to navigate them. This will primarily occur through discussion and direct feedback. Observation of others may be helpful, but be careful. Comparison to others can feel punitive and unhelpful. Remember that any approach you choose is not meant to be a "Gotcha" intervention. You do not want to elicit additional resistance. Be very careful with videotaping if you choose to use this strategy. Interact in a manner that encourages internal motivation.

Questions:
~ How are you going to know that this is a skill you need to develop?
~ What are some pros and cons of choosing to take on the challenge of change?
~ When have you gone through change before?
~ How has previous change come about? What sort of help did you receive?
~ What are the good things about your current situation?, What are the bad things?
~ How do you plan to live independently if...?

Contemplation - Stage 2

If you find your Breakaway to be in the Contemplation Stage, empathy, praise, and support will continue to be important. However, it is now time to more clearly highlight the discrepancies between what they want for themselves and the current behavior they present. It is also time to encourage them to identify possible strategies for overcoming the barriers for change that have been identified. Perceived barriers will become more evident as your encouragement elicits a series of "yes, but" responses and excuses in reply to your questioning.

While not as immediately gratifying as directing and motivating action-oriented behaviors, it is important to remember these efforts will pay off. By intentionally avoiding a confrontation in these early stages, you are acknowledging and letting them grasp their current dilemma of being "stuck" in ambivalence and fear. That acknowledgment is the first step in getting them to experiment with changes in their behavior. It may start with something as simple as a focused effort to get up in the morning, showering daily without reminders, or attending scheduled appointments.

PARENTING STAGE TWO

Developmental Goal:
The goal of this stage is for the developing young adult to identify and examine the benefits and obstacles to change and development.

Strategies:
- Validate their ambivalence, fear, and lack of readiness.
- Encourage the re-evaluation of current behavior. Clarify that the decision about how to change is theirs to make, and assist with the identification of obstacles and behavioral observations.
- Help them to express feelings about the obstacles they face. The expression and acknowledgement of sadness and loss as a result of deficits is important. A frustration for needing to work harder than others, to accept assistance, and to continuously work around obstacles is common. Acknowledging these feelings is an important part of moving forward.
- Encourage exploration of pros and cons of change, and increased awareness of self and current behavior. You want to facilitate the development of a more adult understanding of strengths and weaknesses, an understanding of their own struggles and the impact this has on current behavior and future goals.
- Work toward a positive emotional experience despite adversity. Help them dream of future possibilities, validate frustrations, and assist with the clarification of expectations, goals and direction. Not Action Plans.

Questions:
~ Why is it a good idea to develop these new skills, or to take on added responsibility?
~ How might your life look different a year from now if you learn to _____?
~ How might your life look a year from now if you do not take on the challenge of learning to _____?
~ What are some reasons for keeping things the same? What are reasons to change?
~ What are the things that will make change difficult?
~ What things might be better/worse when you are functioning with independence?
~ What things are getting in the way of the change you need to make?
~ What might help you with taking on this challenge of independence with success?

Preparation - Stage Three

This is the stage where the need for change has been acknowledged and accepted. However they are not necessarily for action. It is the time to more directly encourage progress toward specific action, to highlight the barriers to change, and to identify specific skills and strategies needed to overcome obstacles. ***However, do not push too hard.*** Much ambivalence and uncertainty are likely to still be present. Support, encourage, and establish an expectation for continued development whenever they are ready. The eventual transition to action will occur when these identified skills and strategies are deployed in real world situations, and with less-needed external prompting.

PARENTING STAGE THREE

Developmental Goal:
The goal here is for the Breakaway to get ready for the change that will occur during the next stage. This involves developing the self-determination and greater responsibility. This begins as they experiment with small changes. *Committed action for change however is not the goal.*

Strategies:
- Ask the Breakaway to identify areas of needed growth and areas of strength. This will facilitate the development of confidence and the awareness of strengths.
- Support and reinforce efforts toward growth and development.
- Assist in the identification of obstacles to change, and ways for working over, around, and through these obstacles. Highlight how strengths are useful to overcome obstacles.
- Assist with the identification of available supports.
- Provide assurance that the young adult has the necessary skills for the challenges you have placed in front of them. Encourage small initial steps.

Questions:
~ What makes this change important?
~ How does this change fit into this transition to young adulthood?
~ What might be a good first step in developing the confidence to take this on?
~ Who or what services are available for you to call when you need assistance?
~ During previous times of change, what skills did you use to overcome the anxiety of learning?
~ What areas of struggle do you need to anticipate and plan for in advance?
~ What are some things you might do when experiencing a setback or adversity?
~ Who might you call other than me in the case of an emergency or difficulty at school?
~ You do know that you are ready to do this? Right?

Action - Stage Four

The early "baby steps" of the Action Stage are not always met with instant success and that should not be expected. It is the desire and determination that define this stage and represent a major breakthrough. Even now, as the Breakaway begins to actually break away and become more proactive, an instinctual resistance to change will still rear its head and stall their progress on occasion.

How do you keep maintaining motivation, nurturing the growth of new skills?

PARENTING STAGE FOUR

Developmental Goal:
The goal of this stage is for the young adult to take responsibility for their own development, and the self-determination to follow through with the use of new behaviors.

Strategies:
• Reinforcement of behavior change and efforts toward maintenance. This includes both helping the young adult to recognize and reward their own behavior change, and the use of external rewards provided by you.

• Development of a more mature or adult-to-adult relationship for providing support. Challenges will continue to present themselves, but now is the time to provide assistance that does not recreate a much younger parent-child relationship. The assistance you provide is intended to facilitate the Breakaways effort to take self initiated action and not simply to follow directions. It is also appropriate to connect the developing young adult with a therapist who may provide individual or group supportive counseling.

• Active coaching and instruction for the development of more effective and age-appropriate behavior. Skill development in the areas of organization and time management techniques, relaxation skills, assertiveness and self-advocacy, positive self-talk, and other coping skills. The support of a therapist or coach might be helpful here if you are experiencing resistance. External support is also consistent with desire for greater independence.

• Avoidance of situations that cause problem behavior. It is appropriate to assist in the development of plans to reduce maladaptive behavior related to video game systems, computers, money management, poor sleep and study habits, and isolation. Strategies may include the removal of items, limited access, or minutes allowed.

Questions:
The intent of questions you ask at stage four should be motivated by the goal of developing their sense of self-efficacy and determination. As with questions asked at stage three, normalize and predict struggles, and encourage your young adult to formulate their own responses. At this point you are not only teaching specific skills, but also the ability to adapt to adversity and work around obstacles.

Maintenance - Stage Five

Finally, this is the time for you to provide praise and support, and to elicit thought about success and difficulties. Maintenance of any new behavior requires effort. By discussing the success and difficulties that have occurred, you are encouraging a self-awareness to diligently monitor and sustain the changes made. These new behaviors should hopefully then transfer, apply to other situations in the future.

PARENTING STAGE FIVE

Developmental Goal:
The goal at this stage is to maintain the behaviors and skills that were developed during level four.

Strategies:
- Support and praise the significant efforts that were made during previous stages.
- Acknowledge struggles and efforts to persist and overcome.
- Discuss the potential of Back-Sliding.
- Encourage maintenance of new behaviors and skills until they have become routine.
- Support, support, support when faced with Back-Sliding or regression.

Questions:
Like stage four, the questions of stage five should be motivated by the goal of developing their sense of self-efficacy and determination. Continue to normalize and predict struggles, and encourage your young adult to formulate their own responses. Remember, *you are not only coaching specific skills, you are also coaching the ability to adapt to adversity and work around obstacles. Model these skills for them throughout this process.*

Responding to Push-Back & Resistance

Despite your best efforts there will be Recycling to previous, and less developed behaviors, before forward momentum is re-established. It's just human nature. However, there are several traps to which many unsuspecting parents fall victim, missteps you will want to minimize or avoid altogether if possible.

Trap 1: The Question/Answer Trap

This occurs when parents fall into a pattern of question/answer interactions, where questions are asked as a provocation. Information may be exchanged, but it has little depth or meaning. Sometimes parents may even ask and answer their own questions before a response is possible, with the intention of "making a point", and in hopes of initiating thought or motivation. Neither generally occurs. Instead, this pattern only encourages passivity and compliance in the young adult as they are not challenged to think or engage at a deeper level. In this trap the parent continues to assert their authority, and is very much in charge. For example, *"You know that your brother was doing much more at your age?", "Are you not trying because you are feeling unchallenged (anxious, depressed, overwhelmed, angry etc.)?", "Does your boss just not understand the challenges you face?", "Why don't you just go to class?", "You do know that dad and I are not going to support you forever?", "What is wrong with you?", "When are you going to get it together?", "You are aware that we are not going to continue paying for this support if you don't take advantage of it?".*

If you find yourself caught in this trap, you will want to shift your style of engagement to one that challenges the passivity. Questions should be open-ended (requiring more than a one-word response), and challenging enough to require more than a canned response.

There are two techniques that might be helpful to get out of this rut --

The first technique is referred to as ***What's going great?/What could be better?*** Because while question/answer interactions tend to be problem or task-oriented, the interaction here is intended to be the opposite, as "challenges" or "obstacles" are not discussed. Instead, the focus is shifted to what is going well, and because perfection is an impossibility, those areas that, "could be better". This can be a great way to start a conversation, especially with someone who does not see that anything they are doing is problematic. You will experience less push-back, while you both have an opportunity to explore the positives that do exist. This will help feed the momentum you are seeking.

To initiate this conversation, begin with questions or comments about all that is going well and what they see as strengths. Do not be critical or debate what they perceive as positive if you disagree. Instead, use this interaction to better understand their perspective, to celebrate the positives, and to build rapport. Once they have exhausted all of the positives, take time to summarize and follow-up with questions about what they would like to be better in their lives. More often than not, they will find a few things that could be better. Go slow, but recognize that this shift is a first step toward change.

By having this conversation, a parent is modeling, in a non-threatening manner, the discussion of one's strengths and weaknesses. The Breakaway is taking a risk by exposing their weaknesses, and the parent's role is to encourage this behavior by not attacking, by not jumping-in to fix, or even making suggestions. These interactions are about changing the nature of your relationship and discussions. You are working to reduce push-back and to position yourself more as a coach and less as "the parent". Take time to listen, and allow a stronger relationship to develop.

Another technique for getting out of the Question/Answer trap is called *Looking Back or Reminiscing*. This simply involves having a conversation about all that your Breakaway has experienced prior to this transition into young adulthood. It is a great opportunity to recall successes, failures, and obstacles overcome. Point out times when high levels of support were needed, and times where just simple perseverance made the difference. As the conversation continues, wonder aloud how they might face similar challenges now, but needing much less external support. This awareness of all their ups and downs (all long since survived) and the long journey they have been on, the progress they have made, is pivotal.

Trap 2: The Expert Trap

This occurs when a parent or counselor immediately proceeds to direct the young adult's change and to convince them what must be accomplished, without first considering their readiness or the direction they would like to take. In this situation a parent might say, *"Without better organizational skills (or social skills) you're never going to get anything done. I know someone who can help,"* or *"We really have got to get you eating better"*, *"Do you know that putting on weight like you have, is unhealthy and limits your ability to function at your true potential? I know that you'll feel much better"*. The problem here is that in the face of adult persuasion, the Breakaway often becomes passively compliant to all suggestions/directions made. Only halfhearted efforts are then made as they follow the "expert" leadership provided. Not a great approach for encouraging the developing of autonomy and self-efficacy. Remember, always reference the Stages of Change to facilitate your understanding of their potential receptiveness to your efforts. Change will always occur on their time schedule not yours.

A more effective approach is not one absent of direction, ***but one that offers direction only when the Breakaway's motivation is sufficiently high enough to accept it.*** Accepting assistance from others is most welcome when there has been exploration of multiple alternatives, not before. This provides an opportunity for some mistakes and setbacks, and as a result, the development of sufficient incentive for the risk of change. Ideally, a situation can be created where the young adult feels a sense of control and asks for assistance.

It must be noted, however, there are times when it is not only appropriate, but imperative, for a parent to step in and overrule, regardless of what the Breakaway wants. Issues of safety are the most obvious cases in point. Overall though, parents should strive for fewer and fewer such interventions, and to side-step the "expert trap" whenever possible.

Trap 3: The Labeling Trap

This refers to the tendency of parents to view all behavior through the limited lens of their child's diagnosis, and the desire to have their (now) young adult do the same.

For many, once the diagnosis is official, all effort to understand the impact of age, maturity, personality, or any number of other influences, ceases. The diagnosis trumps all and their child's complex identity is lost. This blanket label is the answer to every question. The excuse, the albatross and the solution, all in one. For example, in response to a complaint about attending a support group, a parent might say, ***"I don't care if you want to go or not. You know your Autism makes it difficult to make friends. You should really go to that social skills group".*** This is a deficit-based response, rooted in the simple formula of: ***Diagnosis = Deficits; Intervention = Less Deficits.***

Simple, right?

Please don't misunderstand me. I'm not saying that such concern is illogical or misguided; just that there is a risk of failing to consider other contributing factors, to not fully see the individual and their situation. It is a lazy shorthand approach. It is also oppressive and dehumanizing to a population still wrestling with the burden of that diagnosis, felt solely as a stigma that marks them, a scarlet "A" tattoo that cannot be washed off.

For this reason it is helpful to use the label of a diagnosis sparingly, while instead referring to observable strengths and weaknesses, or obstacles. In this way you will be addressing the behavior and not the labels, which is very important, given the enormous variability in presenting behavior observed in individuals on the Spectrum, identified as 2e, or a combination of both. ***Don't make the diagnosis the focus, but rather the obstacles that arise from it.***

Trap 4: The Premature Focus Trap

This trap has been discussed throughout the chapter and involves getting too far ahead of the developing young adult in charge of this process. For example, ***"Lets develop an action plan for how you are going to meet more people"***. While it is not effective leadership to simply follow their lead, you must motivate from a position that is relevant and meaningful, based in an understanding for where they are and not where you want them to be. Otherwise you simply won't be heard. Resist the temptation to move too fast. Take time to develop trust and rapport and ultimately a path of least resistance. Sometimes the identification of a clear area of focus can take weeks or months. Continue to encourage them to try new things, to have new experiences, and to challenge themselves. This expands their experience and often creates the opportunity for the Breakaway to identify areas that they are motivated to work on. It also helps to maintain momentum.

Trap 5: The Blaming Trap

When things are not going well, it is a natural tendency for a parent to blame their Breakaway, and conversely, for the Breakaway to blame their parents. ***"If you would just listen…!"***

This is not a productive use of energy and does little to promote forward momentum. Blame should be avoided at all cost. Establish a blame-free culture and model the skills of problem-solving under pressure. If you find yourself being blamed for something, rather than responding in anger, stay calm. Redirect the conversation to one of possibilities and solutions, to next steps, and to calm. The valuable skills for every young adult to have is calm first, then thinking of next steps. If the Breakaway is frustrated it's doubtful that the "teachable moment" you may be seeking is presently occurring. Once they are calm and future focused you may then utilize the experience of this adversity as a teachable moment.

Two Case Studies: Responding to Change

Now, as you read the following case studies, ask yourself where in the Stages of Change model do these kids fall? What strategies are the parents using to identify the stage and promote progression? What traps have the parents fallen into? What might you do differently?

Ron

By all accounts Ron was a bright guy. He was twenty years old, enrolled in college, and arguably, for the first time, had acknowledged the need to find a direction that fit his skills and abilities. Ron, unfortunately, seemed unwilling or unable to take advantage of what was laid out before him. Mostly, he just seemed content to play video games and surf the web for Anime movies and the next convention. Ron was capable of doing the work required to complete his classes, but except for one computer class, he would avoid his assignments unless pushed. It saddened his parents to see this behavior, and that they were apparently unable to help him move on with his life.

In an effort to correct this situation, Ron's parents and his therapist worked to teach him skills of organization and time management. They had set a reinforcement schedule, and had long discussions about the importance of goal-setting and achievement, the impact his diagnosis has on the difficulties he was experiencing, and the need to take charge of his life and future. They helped him establish goals, and were very directive in helping him to reach them. Ron was not always cooperative or happy to see them, but they were sure that this extra push would be the key for turning things around.

Ever since Ron was identified as Twice Exceptional at the age of 12, great efforts had been made to provide support and to help Ron compensate for his weak executive functioning skills and slow process speed. He had been attending individual and group counseling for years, and in large measure, this had been successful. Ron had the knowledge to deploy a great number of these skills to his benefit. He responded well to routine and predictability, and at home demonstrated a willingness to utilize appropriate coping skills on his own. This ability made all the difference in his graduation from high school.

These efforts, however, did not have the same effect now that he was in college and needing to become more independent. Ron was not responding in the same way. Again, this was puzzling since he had already demonstrated the ability to do this, and had great things laid-out for himself. He even had a team of supporters ready to help him take action. Ron's parents were frustrated, and they were increasingly open to taking their friend's suggestion that it was time to cut him off from their support. He just seemed too unmotivated or lazy to justify the energy and resources they were putting into this effort.

At the end of long conversations, Ron would eagerly make a decision about the direction and next steps he would like to take. This pleased his parents, and helped to define the strategy that everyone would be taking. However, Ron never seemed capable of follow-through. The more everyone pushed, the more Ron seemed to resist. This seemed crazy! After all, was not this Ron's desired goal and direction? It was all so puzzling and sad!

Standing back from the situation, it is clear that Ron was not prepared for so much change so soon. While he was genuinely interested in the direction he had chosen in school, he did not fully grasp all that choice entailed, and was not sure he could, or wanted to, leave behind the comfort of his current situation. He was conflicted. More of the same vs. growth, discomfort vs. opportunity. For now, wallowing in the familiar and the safety of well-worn coping skills was his only answer. Ron was still "wishing" for changes. Stalling for time, if you will. He was firmly entrenched in the Contemplation Stage, not ready for action.

Consequently, the support given to him needed to focus more on his awareness of his own behavior, its effectiveness (or lack thereof) within his current circumstance, and the responses it engendered from others. *He needed assistance in evaluating his strengths and weaknesses and their impact on his daily functioning. He needed time to be sad about the obstacles his deficits presented and the limitations he felt. To sort out who he was and what he, in fact, wanted to become.* No longer interested in blindly following whatever adults thought was best for him, Ron wanted to ponder his own future before deciding his way forward.

Stacey

Stacey on the other hand was ready for action. She had already spent a year trying school on her own and struggled greatly. While disappointing, this experience had also proven to be very helpful. Stacey, more than ever before, had an understanding of her areas of weakness and was interested now in receiving coaching to help her in these areas.

Stacey knew that she struggled with organizing her time, and that she struggles to manage the anxiety she experienced daily as part of her Autism Spectrum Disorder. She could articulate when, where and how things fall apart for her, and wanted tips and support to overcome resulting obstacles. She was ready for an approach that was action-oriented. She had the desire and willpower to take charge of these changes. She appreciated the helping relationships she had with tutors, parents and her psychologist, and was even open to a reward system that encouraged the development and maintenance of the behaviors she was working so hard to develop.

Her parents and tutors were also very excited to work with Stacey. Everyone could see great potential, and all were universally excited to see what she would accomplish in her life.

This is why everyone became so frustrated when her commitment seemed to waver. Stacey's grades had slipped, and she seemed satisfied with doing the bare-minimum. Her social life now seemed more important than her goal of a degree and a career. As the semester progressed, Stacey was increasingly late to her tutoring sessions, was often unprepared, and was even known to miss these appointments. Everyone was concerned.

Tensions increased as Stacey's parents became more actively engaged in the planning of her daily schedule. They had not expected to do this, but there seemed to be no other option, as there were legitimate fears that her GPA would drop below a 3.0. Stacey's parents were also concerned about the choices that she was making in her friends. None seemed committed to an education, and their interests seemed more consistent with those of thirteen year-olds than young college women. They were very clearly an unwanted distraction, but her parents were unsure how to respond. This was not the Stacey that they had known when she was at home.

While the support Stacey's parents and tutors were providing was quite appropriate when the semester began, what they failed to recognize was that…

She had regressed from Stage Four all the way back to Stage Two.

Now that she was in this new environment of college, she was not as confident as she had been. She lacked the conviction to charge ahead. It was all so much more challenging than she had anticipated. As a result, she was once again going through the process of contemplating and questioning the changes that would need to be made.

For their part, Stacey's parents and tutors needed to recognize this shift and adjust their approach to fit her needs. They needed to recognize that Recycling or back-sliding is a normal part of the change process, and that her slowed progress would not result in dire consequences.

Ron and Stacey have much in common. Because of this, it is understandable you might try to use a uniform approach of support and encouragement. But they are also two different people and experiencing this transition in their own way, and at their own pace as they move through the stages of change. There is no, and never will be, and specific schedule that must be followed. This must be taken into account by those providing support.

Even as Breakaways graduate to the Action and Maintenance stages, your job as Coach can be just as fraught with stumbling blocks and just as necessary.

Here's an example of a successful resolution at a more advanced stage.

Stewart

Stewart, a twenty year-old diagnosed with ASD, would not consider any support or guidance that did not first recognize his desire for complete independence. He wanted to become a physician's assistant (PA), and he was determined to get there, no matter what it took. He also was tired of being the guy who needed lots of external support. Stewart was conflicted. Shouldn't he be ready to move forward all on his own…? By accepting continued support wouldn't he be acknowledging that he was somehow less than others? He certainly didn't want to sell himself short!

While this was admirable, and while in many ways he had the skill set to achieve this goal, Steward also struggled to fully recognize where his areas of weakness would trip him up at this next level. This had everyone very worried.

He still had more to learn about himself, and the reality of balancing his academic workload while living on his own. He was not yet ready to do this without some external support.

Those supporting him had to walk a fine line. Stewart obviously needed them, but it was apparent a direct, solution-focused approach was not the place to start. That would only lead to power struggles. Instead, those helping Stewart needed to put away the hammer. They needed to listen and be more subtle in their methods. Rather than jumping in with their own agenda, they started by acknowledging his strengths, and desire to be seen as someone capable. Someone not disabled. They listened, and incorporated what they heard into a strategy for moving forward, one that everyone could agree upon.

With this as a basis for future interactions, Stewart became more willing to accept the support he needed.

Stewart felt heard and respected, and subsequently opened up more by sharing his own areas of concern and anxiety. He was beginning to collaborate. While he continued to be guarded, receiving support no longer was perceived as threatening or minimizing. It was simply part of maturing into an independent young man.

Stewart could now acknowledge his areas of weakness and accept support in areas of absolute need. He even became more open to soliciting help in those areas where he was provided more latitude, but had still struggled to find success. This represented a process of learning and understanding on both sides, and the ultimate outcome was very positive.

It was, however, a long process that unfolded over more than a year, made possible only by his parent's astute appraisal of what they were experiencing and observing.

Having reviewed the Stages of Change, try to gauge your Breakaway's readiness. As mentioned previously I recommend writing your answers in a notebook/journal so that you can record and return to your observations, thoughts and feelings at each stage of the process, and get the clarity that one often finds in working out a problem on paper.

Where Do You Stand?

1. Where would you place their overall readiness for this transition on the Stages of Change?
2. In what areas would you place their readiness for change in Stage One or Two?
3. Are there specific behaviors or areas of change that are more reflective of Stages Three, Four, or Five?
4. Where might you expect the most Recycling or Back-Sliding?
5. In what stage do you place your own readiness for the change to come?
6. How is your current approach toward your young adult similar or different from the approaches described above?

Notes

Notes

Expectations

A master can direct you and tell you what he expects.
A teacher, though awakens your own expectations.

Patricia Neal

The Breakaway

The establishment of appropriate expectations, ones sufficiently challenging and realistic, is critical for the emotional and psychological health of a Breakaway.

These expectations will not only shape the manner in which they take on adversity and challenge, but also the internal dialogue that drives the choices they make - especially as it relates to their dreams of the future. For this reason it is important that their development is collaborative. Expectations established unilaterally, only to be presented to the Breakaway, are sure to be met pushback and resistance. Collaboration and buy-in continue to be central to all of your efforts.

Generally, the expectations we place on children and adolescents tend to arise from two very different philosophies, *Performance-Based* and *Learning-Based*. While the intention may be the same, the goals and long-term outcomes of each could not be further apart. Performance-based expectations are all about outcomes. Putting points on the board, ticking boxes, collecting trophies, and no matter what, keeping pace with others. Reduced to its core, it is simply the tracking of behavior and output until the appearance of success has been met.

On the other hand, learning-based expectations are about discovering the *process* needed to achieve desired goals. This approach recognizes the importance of outcomes, of course, but focuses on the many small things needed for them to occur with consistency. Struggle and setbacks are not avoided, but rather understood to be essential, as growth cannot occur if the Breakaway does not learn to step outside of their comfort zone. Setbacks and a slower pace are actually embraced and encouraged as crucial components of sustained growth, as the skills learned through hard earned progress, tend to make future obstacles seem less daunting. This will not occur if established expectations are focused on immediate gratification and success. *Again, the process itself is what matters.*

Performance-based expectations are not inherently bad. It's just that an over-emphasis on performance inadvertently sends a message that outcomes are more important than learning.

Sadly, our current academic climate of standardized testing and score-based salaries for teachers only perpetuates this superficial approach. It has become the dominant methodology in our education system. It has no doubt impacted Breakaways, as external schedules and deadlines better suited for others are imposed on them with great regularity. Everyone involved in their lives is then driven by the pressure to keep up – or at least maintaining the perception of keeping up. For a population notorious for going at their own pace and trajectory, who do not easily break down larger goals into their incremental steps, this makes little sense. It is true those on the receiving end of this approach can learn to adapt. They can be pushed to jump through the hoops. That doesn't mean growth and development are actually being achieved. As with anyone faced with the mounting pressure of deadlines, their focus will turn to getting the job done as quickly and pain-free as possible. Shortcuts are taken, corners cut, and opportunities for growth may even be avoided if they are seen as a potential threat to the external image they want (need!) to project. These kids become very skilled at deflection and evasion. In the short run this facade can be extremely convincing, but the lack of skill development takes a huge toll further down the road.

The bottom line is performance-oriented and Learning-oriented techniques reflect two completely opposite, conflicting belief systems.

Performance people view ability as relatively fixed and unchanging. In other words, you are what you are. Those operating within this fixed mindset do not establish high aspirations for themselves beyond their current ability. The perceived value of their own performance is based on the direct comparison to the expectations and performance of others. They focus more on immediate results than long-term goals and they are less likely to embrace the link between hard work and success, as they have not practiced and built the skill of delayed gratification. Performance people are also more likely to fall in the trap of comparing themselves to others, making it even harder to acknowledge that they need coaching and assistance.

The Learning people, though, view ability as a malleable and tangible quantity that can be developed over time. Thus, hard work and persistence, while uncomfortable, have value. One's position in the world, skill level and intelligence can be grown. Nothing is fixed. Individual effort is real and every observed success is achievable.

Most of my students, at least in the beginning, have the former world view. If they can't immediately master some material, they are not inclined to waste time trying. They cover with excuses like *"That's too hard for someone with my ability..."*, *"It's boring"*, *"I just don't like that subject"*, or even *"It's not challenging enough"*. **They have not been gifted with the expectation that it is possible to take on big challenges if they are met with equally big efforts.**

Once they have that new outlook, they are more eager to take on new and challenging tasks. They remain engaged in the learning process despite the discomfort, and in spite of the fact others can see that they do not yet know what they are doing. Not surprisingly, their performance continues to improve, because...well, it's a possibility now.

Interestingly enough, when experiencing success, learning-oriented and performance- oriented individuals are virtually indistinguishable. They both display positive attitudes, and are both successful at deploying different strategies to overcome challenges. However, as soon as significant adversity is introduced into the equation, these opposite profiles emerge.

Learning-oriented individuals increase their efforts, continue to deploy new strategies, and are able to improve their performance. They know it will take longer and require more effort and work than their neurotypical peers. They also have the abiding faith that with dedication they will learn it. The performance-oriented individual is not able to do this. Instead, their attitude turns increasingly negative, with an overall deterioration in performance, and limited use of problem-solving strategies.

To illustrate this further, let us look at the example of Josh and Neal as they transition to life after high school.

Josh & Neal: 2 Belief Systems

Both Josh and Neal struggled with obstacles related to their Twice Exceptional classifications. Both were excited about the prospects of the new adventures they would have as they enrolled at the local community college. Both had an awareness of their deficits, and acknowledged additional support and coaching would be necessary as they adjusted to greater independence.

Josh came from a background where his parents were Performance-oriented, where the mastery and development of skills was highly praised and valued. They helped Josh establish goals and celebrated greatly when each was achieved. Determined that he would fit in as well as his siblings did at school, they chose to downplay his deficits and highlight his achievements. The goal was to build up Josh's sense of what was possible. But ironically, when faced with such high expectations and enumerable setbacks compared to his siblings and peers, Josh had been "taught" the reverse: he had severe limitations and they were unlikely to change no matter what he did.

Rather than having his efforts reinforced, Josh had learned to let others help him beyond what he really needed, continually compared himself to others, and played exclusively to his strengths to avoid areas of weakness. When unable to obtain positive affirmation, anxiety and frustration, followed by helplessness and avoidance, set in. Achievement had been reinforced, not effort. He thus avoided those tasks that would not provide immediate positive reinforcement, or at worst might result in shame.

From his perspective, the struggle of learning at a slower pace, with limited chance of positive returns, made little sense. However, when others focused on his strengths while glossing over and accommodating his deficits, Josh felt great. To Josh and his parents this was a sign of "normality" – finding external rewards without the discomfort of growth was a lot more fun.

Neal's background was different. He came from a family where achievement was also important, but where effort and attempts to solve problems were praised first. His family normalized frustration and discomfort, encouraging it actually. They did not ignore the mastery of skills, as they were highly celebrated and expected, but this was not their main focus of attention. Instead, they came to expect struggle, and praised his efforts to work over, around or through obstacles when they presented themselves. They wanted Neal to approach the world as a person who both expects and takes on challenges. Rather than working toward finish lines, they wanted him to have a "what's next" mentality as he moved through life.

This is where he focused his energy. He had learned to ask the questions: "How can I do it?", "What will I learn?", "What are the worst things that could happen?", "What is the best thing that could happen?", "What's the most likely thing to happen?", and "What should I do next?". He understood the answers to these questions may not always be easy, but that was okay. He was not afraid to let others see him struggle.

Progression through school and task-completion was secondary to having Neal experience the struggle and reward of learning. While his parents had expectations that he do well, they were not prone to writing his papers, and would not do his homework just to get it completed. Work was not always as well-done as his parents might have liked, but it was completed. As a result, Neal tended to run a quarter to a semester behind each year, and it took him longer to graduate high school.

Both families helped their boys graduate with the basic skills needed for greater independence, with approximately the same level of ability in most areas.

Josh & Neal Meet Adversity

At the time of their enrollment in college, the academic placement test identified some significant deficits for both Josh and Neal in the area of Arithmetic. As a result, they were both placed in a developmental or pre-college level math class that met each day. Its goal was to establish the math skills necessary for higher level college classes. This was the very same goal that Josh and Neal established for themselves.

The teacher, being aware of each student's history of frustration with math, wanted to first practice those skills they had already mastered. She wanted to reinforce this learning and instill confidence before moving on to more challenging work.

Both thrived in this environment. They showed an interest in coming to tutoring and enjoyed the tasks they were given. They even supported one another through verbal encouragement and peer tutoring. Things were going very well, and they were actually having fun.

After four weeks of this practice and reinforcement, the teacher decided it was time to introduce more difficult math problems. What occurred next is very interesting. Despite his obvious frustration of multiple failures, Neal persisted. He remained positive about the task, and was even able to joke about how hard things had become. He had energy for the task ahead. He was enjoying the challenge of learning. And, with time he showed incremental improvement. Progress was slow, but his tutor was confident he would be ready for college level math within a semester, maybe two.

By contrast, Josh had become rather pessimistic. Frustrated by his struggles, he had become less energized, more distracted, and required much redirection to keep on task. He was no longer smiling like he once had, and was not interested in receiving support from Neal. His efforts to learn the material had become halfhearted and sloppy. He became more oppositional, would say he didn't care, was cheating to get the result he wanted, and began to ditch class all together.

Feeling unable to master the new skills as quickly as Neal, he felt stupid. "I should know this!"; "If they would just put me in the regular class I would do better."; "This teacher is terrible and doesn't like me."; "I just don't take placement tests well."; "I've alreadydone this math."; "This is BS!"; I'm not a SPED kid..."; and "This sucks!", were now common themes for Josh.

When informed of the situation, Josh's parents first responded by questioning the quality of instruction he was receiving and directed their anger toward the teacher and her approach. After all, he had received high marks in his high school math classes. When it became clear his teachers were not the problem, they became mad at Josh. Threats were made and new performance goals were established.

Poor Josh had never learned the skill of fighting through frustration to find success, and so could not deploy this skill now that he was on his own.

Learning, skill-development, and mastery of anything is not a process of immediate gratification. There is always a necessary period of failure, confusion, and discomfort, and there are never any guarantees for any outcome. It cannot be avoided.

With their expectation of only "winning" dashed, both Josh and his parents had a very long academic year ahead of them.

Fortunately, they were ultimately willing to seek the assistance of support professionals who helped them understand Josh's current developmental needs and skill deficits. This resulted in a new approach that more specifically reinforced exploration, rather than the simple achievement of defined goals. Not surprisingly, with this shift Josh began to thrive. It took time, but he became more willing to accept support, and to let others see that he was struggling.

Once they all had learned that struggle was inevitable and "normal" and not a crisis requiring an immediate change in direction, the fear and anxiety dropped significantly. Effort, resiliency, and a willingness to ask for help took their place.

The example of Josh and Neal very clearly illustrates how parental expectations and reinforcement can influence the development of a world-view that enables one to find success despite the presence of obstacles.

Neal did not develop his coping skills and persistence by accident.

They were the natural outgrowth of his parents' expectations – their reinforcement and relaxation about the process radiated a feeling of *eventual success* and encouraged Neal to be honest about where he was in his learning. Essentially, he had nothing to lose.

Josh's parents, meanwhile, radiated fear of failure. They projected this fear onto Josh, and those expectations taught Josh to lie and pretend if necessary to continue receiving their approval. His parents were determined he not be "limited" by his diagnosis, and yet their own panic became his biggest handicap and impediment to success.

This did more damage to his self-esteem than any failure might have.

Neal's parents knew that many things were going to be difficult in Neal's life, and wanted to establish a work ethic that would give him the wherewithal to face them all down.

If you find yourself identifying more with the approach taken by Josh's parents, don't worry. It is not too late to tweak your approach. To establish expectations that acknowledge and even embrace discomfort. For many this represents an entirely new way of operating, the adjustment may take some time. However, if the expectation you set for your Breakaway is the development of perseverance…you need only take a deep breath and lead by example.

Expectations in Action

In conclusion, it is important to set expectations that are both learning and performance-based, but most especially ***Reality-based***. Expectations beyond the Breakaway's ability to achieve them, will erode their trust in you, and significantly slow progress. Early performance feedback should reward and encourage, but always emphasize effort or progress over specific achievements. ***At all times, struggle and anxiety should be normalized. Even the slightest bit of momentum should acknowledged.*** More definitive, clear-cut benchmarks can be established later on, when forward momentum has been observed with greater consistency.

By anticipating the reality of the struggle to come, your responses to situations will become more measured and intentional, less likely to be based in fear or anger. Focus on your young adult regaining their equilibrium whenever buffeted by this bumpy transition period and not losing faith or their vision of what they want. That's what matters most.

As a parent, it is often difficult to maintain objectivity. Opinions will naturally be affected by the love for your child, the potential you see and hope for, and the behavior you have observed all their life. Find professionals in your area with an expertise in Autism Spectrum and 2e profiles and get their perspective. Remember, you do not have to act alone in making these decisions about next steps.

First, I'd like you to begin by ***identifying your expectations as they stand right now.*** And I ask you to be completely – even brutally – honest with yourself.

Please take a moment to write down your thoughts, hopes, fears and expectations for what is to come next. This is an important starting place. Please encourage your spouse or partner to independently do the same. Agreement between parents at this point is not expected, although eventual agreement will be important. For now, just start writing.

I have included examples below from parents with whom I have previously worked. However, please don't confine your answers to the content of the examples listed. This exercise is about you and your experience, not a specific format. However you choose to work out your thoughts and feelings on paper, it's all appropriate.

41

Examples of Parent Expectations & Fears

- We're not worried. Our daughter will develop the skills she needs and will find her place in the world.

- I would love my son to achieve independence, but I expect that we will need to provide continued support.

- I am not sure what to expect for my child after high school. It is overwhelming when I even think about next steps. Mostly anxiety.

- I really don't think may child can do it, but he has convinced us that he should be allowed to try.

- We have taught our son the skills of independence, but are aware it will not be easy for her.

- I have always been told that my daughter will not live with independence, but I know it is possible.

- I am terrified for my son as he faces the challenges of the world alone.

- My son is not capable of transitioning to higher levels of independence. We (parents and siblings) will be providing support in the form of housing and finances forever.

- I'm not sure if I am ready to let my child face the world without our support.

- What you are talking about does not fit our situation. Our son's skills are beyond those of others discussed here. We do not expect to be that involved after he goes off to college.

- We are expecting that our daughter will be going to college, and we expect to relocate to provide the support she needs.

To expand your awareness even further, here is a quiz designed to identify talking points and facilitate a discussion about expectations.

Expectations Quiz

On a single piece of paper, write your answers to the following questions about the expectations and plan you are hoping to establish for your Breakaway's upcoming transition into a life of greater independence.

1. What skills must they develop if they are to be successful in this next stage of life?
2. Given what you know about strengths and weaknesses, what are your immediate expectations for them after high school?
3. What are your long-term expectations for them as they mature into adulthood?
4. How do you define a successful transition?
5. How do you define success in the long-term?
6. In what areas do you expect to see success?
7. What areas do you expect to see difficulty?
8. How do you expect them to respond to setbacks, adversity, and failure?
9. How will you respond to setbacks, challenges and failure?
10. What level and type of support do you see them needing as they make this transition?
11. What support do you expect them to need throughout their life?
12. What steps do you need to take to assure that the appropriate level of support will be in place?
13. What level of independence do you expect them to have in the area of money management?
14. What is a reasonable budget?
15. Assuming they are living in their own apartment, what are your expectations for the apartment's appearance and general cleanliness?
16. What is most important to you during this time of transition?
17. As your role as a parent transitions to one of less involvement, how will you fill the extra time you now have?
18. Would you describe your current style of parenting as one based in Control, or one based in Influence? Which best fits the style of your spouse?
19. How do you expect to monitor your own performance as a parent, leader, and guide?
20. How do you think your responses would compare to those of your young adult's, teachers, therapist, tutors, etc.?

Six Key Points To Remember

1. Expectations should be reality-based. Expectations that are set too high or two low are counterproductive to further development.

2. Remember, expectations will be communicated through both your words and your nonverbal behavior. Be mindful of the messages you are sending. How you choose to respond to their choices will shape their behavior and advancement. Respond, but don't overreact.

3. Identify your own private expectations, be honest with yourself. Take time to identify the expectations you have already established. Evaluate their appropriateness for your current situation. Seek guidance. An outside opinion from a professional can be invaluable.

4. Understand it is impossible to control everything. Give yourself permission to "lose control", and for your aspiring young adult to make mistakes. This will not be easy, but will become easier as you let go of the stress that comes with needing to control everything.

5. Create a ladder of well-defined steps/outcomes. If you develop a long-range plan, a structure to work within, your fears will lose their strength. Success and adversity on a daily basis will have context, you will judge less and focus more on how they relate to the goal. Changes to short-term and intermediate goals will then be based strategic planning rather than fear and impulse.

6. Prioritize. It is not possible to make everything happen at once, so stop trying. Take the ladder one step at a time. Learn, breathe and radiate patience. It will be contagious. Your Breakaway needs a steady and unflappable coach – one with a calm understanding of what they are facing and a clear view at all times of the bigger picture. Are you ready to make the changes in yourself as you approach this transition?

44

Notes

The Human Experience

Judge a man by his questions rather than his answer.

Voltaire

The Breakaway

The Human Experience, with not only its variety, but also its nuance, ambivalence, and insecurity, applies just as equally to parents as it does to kids.

Parents who feel great pressure to be perfect – and fall short, as we all do.

As I say, I have had the opportunity to sit with hundreds of Breakaways and their parents, and, trust me, there are always more questions than definitive answers.

Even the answers result in more questions!

The families are usually well-informed and mentally prepared for all this change, but they still struggle to deal with its daily dilemmas and emotions. As one parent told me, *"It's like the pitching machine went from slow to fast-pitch overnight. And we haven't caught up!"*

It can be terrifying, exhilarating, heartbreaking, gratifying, and confusing all at once. Which makes it very tempting to grab for easy fixes and guarantees, some kind of certainty; but ironically, these quick solutions will only cause you more anxiety and stress over time.

The only rule that never changes is:

An effective plan cannot be developed in a crisis.

I, too, have struggled to fight the impulse to jump into "fix-it" mode, or to throw poorly thought-out solutions at problems that were not clearly understood. This was especially true early in my career when I was first starting work with this population. I felt pressure from all sides (including my own) to "make this happen," to live up to everyone's urgent hopes, and quite honestly, to find immediate success.

I felt stuck, and experienced a terrible self-doubt. Was I up to this job?

It was not until a conversation with a very wise parent that I learned how to ask the right questions – ones that took in the bigger (human) picture.

Learning to Ask the Right Questions

At the time I met this particular mother, **Jan**, I was running a weekly support group for parents where we discussed many of the issues covered in this book.

Jan was one of the regular attendees, and my first impression was she must be quite overwhelmed, as she tended to be more of a listener/observer than active participant. In contrast to Jan, our group was comprised mostly of big personalities who processed their experience through lots of animated conversation and vigorous debate. All of them struggling to keep up with the challenges of parenting a special-needs child.

While the topics varied, discussions tended to always find their way back to an underlying tension that had developed between two sets of parents. One group was wholly focused on problem remediation, and had personal styles that were very task-oriented and achievement-based. Collectively, this set of parents was driven by the desire to have their children catch up to their same-age peers.

The other set of parents rejected this view, felt the opposite way. Their perspective was one of unconditional acceptance, an open rejection of any approach driven by the desire to push and build toward "success". Instead, their approach was to support and encourage without pushing. They had also given up on any idea of specific destinations when it came to their children's growth and development.

As close as the entire group of parents had become, there were times when the conversation became heated as imperatives such as "must" and "should" were thrown about. They were all quite passionate and wanted the best for their children. It was clear there were feelings of guilt, fear, and anxiety on both sides, and everyone was trying to do what they thought was correct. They were also working hard to defend their respective approaches and convert others to join their side. They needed reassurance that they were not doing the wrong thing. So the disagreement of others, or worse yet, the success of a different approach, only magnified everyone's insecurities. The tension in the room was high, and I was feeling loads of pressure as the group looked to me to take sides and provide answers.

One evening during a particularly lively debate, Jan, the quiet but regular attendee to the group, raised her hand. What she said entirely changed the direction of the evening discussion - and my perspective on the work I do with this population.

She began by sharing her frustration with parents, teachers, and counselors whose approach to assisting her son had little to do with his needs, and who were always questioning her understanding for the type of support he needed.

Then, it all came spilling out:

They rarely spend the time to get to know me or my son, instead relying on canned IEP goals and interventions - which they never follow through with anyhow. They seem more motivated by their own need to feel helpful and to avoid the appearance that they do not have answers, than they are in helping me and my son get unstuck.

Parents I talk with also seem to be caught in their own trap. Wanting to be helpful and to feel useful, but unsure what the hell to do. Comparison to others seems to be their only measure of success, even when they are trying to be supportive. It has never felt supportive, and in my estimation, it has never been helpful. No offense... I fell into this trap myself.

Every time another parent would brag about their child's success at school, about their improved social development, or their response to some new approach, my heart would ache. And every time I went to a conference to listen to the stories of adults who had succeeded despite their autism, my experience was the same. I felt sick. I knew my son was working hard, but I couldn't let go of the idea that I was a failure, that our approach was wrong, or maybe, that my son still wasn't working hard enough! So then, I would push harder, and harder, despite the uneasy feeling I had doing that.

I understand where you are all coming from. I have been on both sides of the Fix or Don't Fix-It debate, and neither is an easy place to be.

It was hard. Primarily my husband and I were in Fix-It mode. I had based my expectations on what I saw others doing, or the benchmarks other parent's children had achieved. I can't do that anymore. While there is nothing wrong with having expectations for growth, an evaluation process that looks to others as a measurement of success, or that was designed for another, is destined to be miserable. This is what happened to me.

Report card day, IEP meetings, and parent teacher conferences were always a disaster. And yes, our son had come to see our love for him as conditional. Based upon his achievement of the goals we had established. This had become our focus, and thus his main source of praise, attention and esteem. The killer was that with the expectations we had established, he faced more frustrations and failures, than successes.

Unfortunately, the attention he depended upon to feel loved was limited. Our focus was instead directed toward the next innovative strategy, with hopes that these struggles would go away. For my son to find "success". Clearly our priorities were out-of-whack. With the best of intentions, we set him up to fail, and had sent a message that his self-worth was based upon his ability to meet expectations originally developed for another person.

When we were in the "Don't Fix-It mode", it was a time-out of sheer exhaustion, when we just stopped trying. While this felt good to some degree, what we were doing (or rather not doing), also did not feel right. In the end we would overreact to these feelings, becoming even more focused on finding a fix. It was a roller coaster for everyone.

I want my son to know there is nothing more he can do that would make us love him more. Period. That being said, I want him to learn that he has both strengths and weaknesses, and with hard work he can learn to tap into his strengths and minimize his weaknesses.

I do not want my son's life defined by the pursuit and attainment of a "success" designed for others, or for him to be defined by his diagnosis. Rather I want his life to be defined by the pursuit of challenges that are appropriate for his specific skill set. This is what will result in his happiness, and ultimately his independence.

I am wondering if some of you need to reevaluate the way you have come to see this problem of autism? My husband and I saw it as a problem to fix, even as a competition with ourselves and others, and so were not asking the right questions. It's not a competition, a simple case of remediating gaps in development, or a condition to passively accept. Our questions and research based in this framework were not helping us find what we really needed. We were in a negative feedback loop and didn't know it. I wonder if you find yourself doing the same thing. It was true for me, and to some degree is something I fight myself from falling into on a daily basis.

I would give my life to take away the struggles my son is facing, but I can't.

All I am left with, then, is the challenge of understanding, and the task of pushing in a manner that works for HIM.

When she was done, the whole group seemed affected by her words.

Telling her story so sincerely, as someone who had learned some very tough lessons, Jan had encouraged the group to rethink or reframe their endless debate.

She finished by saying that carrying around the baggage of so many "shoulds" and "musts", internalizing and letting them cripple you, was not helping anyone.

After a few moments of thoughtful silence, another parent spoke up: *"How is my kid ever going to be independent if I don't set high enough expectations so he develops the skills needed to make that happen?"* Another said, *"I will not have my kid use his diagnosis as an excuse. I don't want to set him up to be living with me forever!"* A third, *"I agree with what you said, but how do I push or encourage my daughter? I need others to show me the right way."*

The discussion then continued along this line of thinking. Inspired by these questions, and through the sharing of their own complex stories as parents of children with disabilities, the conversation shifted away from the extreme poles of "Fix-It" or "Accept-It" to a middle ground focused on those elusive, overlooked human factors. We discussed expectations, both healthy and burdensome, Black-And-White and more relaxed/realistic.

We were now asking very different questions – and for the first time, developing strategies that fit.

For some parents this meant letting go of aspirations for complete independence, while for others, a realization that perhaps their expectations were not set high enough.

Jan had broken the code. She helped the others recognize their shared experience and inevitable differences were not at odds with each other. No rules were hard and fast. Nobody right or wrong. Each "case study" was a child, beautifully complex and multidimensional. They only needed to let go of the pursuit of perfection and take the time to thoroughly appreciate their own circumstances before proceeding.

And, of course, the "leader" of the group, had learned the most of all.

How to ask the right questions…

And when to just shut up.

Getting Started

Listed below are a sampling of talking points and questions that I use with parents. Take some time to consider, and, if you want, answer them honestly with a written response.

Write down whatever you think and feel. There are no correct responses, just increased self-awareness and understanding. Many of these questions will likely spawn additional questions or even seem unanswerable. This is intentional.

Beginning Questions

1. Other than diagnosis, what else might influence your developing young adult's progress into transition?
2. Where are you feeling resistance right now?
3. What is your Breakaway responding best at this time?
4. Are there physical, developmental, medical issues we have not discussed?
5. Are there medical, psychiatric or substance abuse issues, or other stressors in the family?
6. Describe what role each member currently has within your family. How might these need to change with this impending transition?
7. Are you ready to make the changes in yourself as you approach this transition?
8. Are you and your spouse (support team) in agreement with the approach you should take?
9. What supports are available to provide assistance?
10. Are current expectations in line with existing skill sets?
11. Would your developing young adult respond to any of these questions differently?

Resilience

Nobody realizes that some people expend tremendous energy merely to be normal.

Albert Camus

The Breakaway

Do you remember the first time you met your in-laws? What about your first job interview, first date, your first speech, or even your first day at a new job? Do you remember the anxiety you experienced? More importantly, how drained you felt once you were back home, or in more familiar surroundings?

These experiences were both exciting and exhausting – not because they were beyond what you were capable of doing, but rather, because they required a more deliberate and attentive approach: an intense minute-to-minute focus on how you were behaving, what you were saying, every move you made. It simply took more energy to look and act natural. And, while you may have successfully navigated a social or professional minefield, there was in fact nothing natural about it. This type of self-regulation, in many ways, mirrors the daily experience of those identified as ASD or 2e, whose constant battle to appear "normal" leaves them completely drained of energy at day's end, sometimes even sooner.

Self-regulation, sometimes referred to as **Executive Control**, is the act of attending to and controlling behavior, thoughts, emotions and desires. It is something we do on an ongoing basis, and is essential to the ability to start and complete tasks, to plan, to delay gratification, to make decisions, and to modify behavior to fit our surroundings. This process is, of course, quite tiring, especially when we're faced with unfamiliar situations where our behavior and decision-making are not well-practiced and demand a sustained effort. This high level of concentration consumes a great deal of energy, and just like automobiles, we all have a limited amount of internal reserves to fuel us on a daily basis.

And when those reserves are gone, they're gone.

Limited reserves can pose a serious problem for neurodiverse kids. Their presenting deficits necessitate a high rate of fuel consumption and a tendency to use up those internal reserves well before their same-age peers. More so, they are not equipped with the skills needed to recognize when they are "running low," how to conserve energy, or effective strategies for "refueling". Each of these skills are central to problem-solving, combats the impulse to avoid or blame others. Add on the challenges of the "grown-up" world suddenly demanding and pushing for immediate results, and the ability to conserve energy or compensate when feeling diminished is enormously important to one's overall functioning.

All parents and support providers must recognize the more intensely Breakaways focus on skill development and refinement, the less able they are at sustaining these efforts, and their ability to maintain adaptive behavior will become inconsistent.

One always has to be watching for the signs of a system overload.

It is very common for those supporting this population to ask questions like:

Shouldn't things be getting easier as they develop more skills? How is it they were doing so well yesterday, last week or last year, only to be such a disaster today? Maybe they need more opportunities to practice these skills? Maybe they need more tutoring? Maybe I need to be doing more? Maybe all of this is just too much for them? Maybe they just don't care?

When the drop-off in performance is interpreted as a sign of rebellion or laziness, it is all too easy to respond in kind with anger and frustration, slip into crisis mode, push back too hard and the negative feedback loop just continues. What is needed instead is a true and empathetic understanding of the extreme toll paid by these kids as they work to maintain the illusion their "normal" behavior comes easy and natural.

Tuning In

Skeptical parents believe poor motivation is the sole root of low achievement and a greater sense of individual responsibility the simple answer. "The time for using deficits as an excuse not to try is over..." is a common refrain. After all, they say, everyone feels tired after hard work, it's no reason for inappropriate behavior or for not giving a sincere effort. For many, limited reserves, known to psychologists as ***Resource Depletion***, does not feel tangible. It is difficult to measure and thus sounds like one more therapeutic label, of which they have already heard too many. The truth, however, is this is a very real phenomenon that has been studied for quite some time. Interestingly enough, the research has been conducted primarily on neurotypical undergraduate college students, making the comparison to the population we are discussing especially meaningful.

The collective findings have consistently shown that any act of self-regulation – difficult decision-making, new and unfamiliar situations, exercising willpower to not engage in a certain activity, or just monitoring posture and eye contact in social situations – is enough to deplete internal resources sufficiently to influence performance.

Again, these results were observed in a neurotypical population functioning at a high level. In each case, those engaging in these tasks showed a significantly diminished ability to engage in subsequent acts of self-regulation. This included a decreased capacity for impulse control, to complete a focused effort, or to employ any forethought or planning. Quite simply, these "normal" young adults were less effective and more easily distracted by TV, gaming and the internet, as they worked to complete academic assignments. Also, there were measurable decreases in the ability to accurately perceive the passage of time (time at work felt much longer), in physical stamina, pain tolerance, and working memory. There was a reduced capacity for flexibility in reasoning and a diminished ability to persist in the face of failure.

Even simple tasks of daily living were more problematic.

Only after an extended period of rest did performance on these tasks return to the original baseline level.

The impact of these results is exponential when applied to a neurodivergent population. The self-regulation of facial expression, personal appearance, posture, movement, conversation and mood, is expected when they enter the social world of others – when they choose to join "the party". It all requires greater internal resources that will not be available for other tasks of self-regulation. What remains then is an individual who is finding it increasingly difficult to process information quickly and accurately, and who is struggling to keep themselves organized and on-task. As a result, they will reach a point of diminishing returns, especially when what they are doing does not include some level of routine, nor can be mastered through a rule-based approach.

To illustrate the magnitude of their daily challenge, listed below is just a sampling of the questions I know many of these young adults confront at the start of each day. Until "decided" and integrated into the automatic routine and flow of their day, each represents a moment where self-regulation is required and internal resources consumed. These decision thoughts are also often experienced in rapid succession as they are presented below. Try reading this list rapidly and imagine how hard it might be to slow down enough to resolve any of these question. Where might you start?

Should I get up this morning?; Shower or no shower?; Why do I have so much trouble getting to sleep at night?; What if I slept for just a little longer?; Are these clean or dirty?; Should I take my meds?; Where are my meds?; Did I take my meds?; Breakfast?; Wait. Am I still taking meds?; When am I to be at work/school?; If my roommate is not going, why should I go?; Should I go, even though I may be getting sick?; What if the teacher asks me why I missed the last class?; Should I load the dishwasher now or just wait?; What was my work schedule?; Did I ever get my laundry out of the dryer?; Where are my keys?; Is my roommate mad at me?; Where is the cell phone?; What bus do I take again?; Do I have time to play on the computer before I go?; Where did I park the car?; Is everything in my backpack?; What day is it?; Where am I going and how do I get there?; Do I need a jacket?; Should I say hello to my coworkers or go straight to work?; Where should I sit in class?; What am I supposed to be doing again?; Did I brush my teeth?; What was that guy's name?; Did I bring my homework?; Where's my schedule?; Did I say something wrong?; What am I supposed to be doing?; What should I do next?

While you may have noticed that it is tiring simply reading this long list, the significance of these questions lie not only in their sheer number, but also in the reality many of these behaviors do not come naturally to them. Can it be so surprising their temptation is to ignore and avoid? And when learning in one situation does not always transfer to other similar situations, the questions and problems to confront can feel endless.

This is their reality.

A reality we must all come to acknowledge and accept.

Although Resource Depletion is just one among many elements that will influence progress through this transition, ***one can be sure it will have a compounding effect on every situation.*** It can lead to a serious paralysis and inability to advocate for additional support. Skills mastered long ago can suddenly go missing. Even if your son or daughter does not struggle so obviously, at some point they will likely communicate that they cannot or do not want to push forward with what others expect of them. Your job is to be in-tune with the signals they are sending and spot the real issue, so you can tailor expectations and encouragement accordingly.

If the mental energy expended by these kids before 10 a.m. equals the total daily expenditure of a neurotypical young adult, then their ability to maintain forward momentum throughout the day constitutes an epic feat of self-control.

Keep this in mind before promoting more tutoring, longer hours and harder work may not always be a good idea. While you may be feeling the pressure for faster progress, it is essential you stay in sync with their current pace, their ability to keep up.

Skill development is of no use if your Breakaway is too stressed and over-scheduled to utilize the information.

Building Resiliency

So, if every step forward into new experiences, skill development, and independence, causes a step backward, yet another setback, how does one ever get anywhere? You would be forgiven for asking: What is the point? What is the remedy?

The answer can be found in the methodology proposed in every book on physical fitness training. ***Rend, recover, and repeat. The process of tearing and rebuilding.***

Much like a muscle's response to exercise, when one's ability to manage life's pressures is challenged and pushed to fatigue, and then is allowed the correct amount of rest, that ability will respond by getting stronger, more resilient. Each mistake and its learned consequences will improve the individual's endurance. Because just like in the process of becoming physically fit, the act of building stamina is more important than the immediate outcome.

Just as we have been discussing…

Failure is necessary. Failure is training.

This process of being challenged in a deliberate manner, and pushed to go a little further than one thought was possible, creates the capacity to take that "next step" in the future with greater ease. Presented with escalating tests and expectations within a controlled environment, a Breakaway is asked to squarely face their anxiety about each task and work through it, rather than avoiding or quitting. Support is provided, but stressors are not ignored or mitigated to prevent discomfort; they are embraced, and held up as an opportunity to build resilience. This structured approach makes all the difference. It results in improved morale, greater stamina, and lower overall stress levels.

I see this every year with the students I support through this transition. If willing to engage in this process of challenge, fatigue and recovery, great progress always follows. For it is the ability to persevere, more than any IQ score, which determines what one is truly capable of achieving. *Nurturing resilience is the key, not giftedness or inherent talent.*

It bears repeating: unlike their school career up until now, the goal is no longer just good test scores and advancement to the next grade; now the goals are skill-building, autonomy, self-advocacy and self-sufficiency.

The Zone Of Maximum Adaptability

If finding a balance between energy depletion and conservation is the cornerstone of all great coaching, you must come to understand *The Zone Of Maximum Adaptability*.

It's a mouthful, I know. It sounds like a Buddhist meditation technique or something from a football playbook. But this particular Zone is defined as *that range of functioning where an individual's performance is most fluid – where their ability to shift gears and think quickly is functioning at the highest level.* This occurs when the individual has been challenged at a level sufficient to promote maximum effort and focus, without being overloaded. It is based on the idea that performance increases with physical and mental arousal, but that there is an effective range in which individuals can be challenged and stressed, and pushed. This is a zone where learning, development, and performance is maximized - it is here that learning occurs, despite the stress they are experiencing.

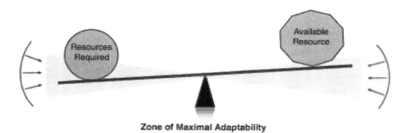

Zone of Maximal Adaptability

Performance drops off sharply when the developing young adult is forced to function outside this range; when individuals become overwhelmed and overloaded, or when they are underestimated and under-challenged. Learning to find this ideal balance will require ongoing and vigilant experimentation. Creating situations and a general atmosphere that keeps your Breakaway "in the zone" as much as possible. They must be pushed and prodded to grow, but at a level that is appropriate to their unique skills and abilities. Too much or too little pushing will create imbalance, a sharp drop-off in their effort and performance.

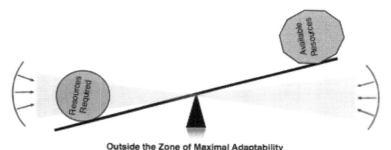

Outside the Zone of Maximal Adaptability

Skills that are well-practiced or have become routine are the least taxing on internal resources. They don't take much thought or concentration to perform. However, as skills become less well-practiced or unfamiliar, energy consumption becomes greater. As a result it is difficult to sustain an effective effort, when faced with a disproportionate number of energy-consuming challenges. Things will very quickly come crashing out of balance, and it is this we are trying to avoid. This population are constantly engaged in emotionally taxing interactions. Often they are simply in survival mode, operating on emergency reserves. Too much time at this extreme level of effort will result in decreased adaptability and resilience.

Breakaways will not always have the language or desire to tell you when they are overwhelmed, or may act in a manner that suggests they just don't care. But when evaluating their behavior, always consider the role this balance may be playing.

Strategies for Balance

When helping parents develop a strategy for finding this elusive balance, The Zone Of Maximum Adaptability, I try to break down skills into four categories from least to most difficult so that one can always keep track of the internal resources being used and used up:

1) Knowing, Doing, & Maintaining: This first category consists of those behaviors or skills, which, for the most part, are already occurring spontaneously. The Breakaway knows how and when to deploy them, can do so with minimal support, and can follow through without any badgering.   There is little instruction here other than rare prompts, continued reinforcement.

2) Knowing/Doing with Prompts and Support: Skills and behaviors here are those for which the Breakaway can describe the reasons they are important, and when and how to deploy them, but for whatever reason, is not able to follow through with regularity or consistency. Frequent prompting and reminders are still very much needed. This might include showering each day, maintaining appropriate eye contact, wearing clean clothes, or brushing one's teeth.

3) Knowing/Learning To Do with Much Support: This category includes skills and behaviors the developing young adult has some working knowledge of, but not at a level that suggests an understanding for when, why, and how they should be used. This might include the use of tools (watch, alarms, calendar etc.) to assure being on-time for class or work, preparing one's own meals, keeping an organized backpack, grocery shopping, staying on budget, maintaining a clean apartment at "young adult standards". Skill development in this area is really pushing the envelope of their comfort zone. These are not necessarily behaviors they see the need for developing, and avoidance or letting others do it for them are typical. Much instruction and motivational "pushing" is required from the coach.

4) Limited Knowledge and Doing Skills: Behaviors in this area are almost entirely new. Either because they are newly needed in this more adult environment, or because the young adult has never been challenged to develop them. Either way, the developing young adult will be starting from square one. Much instruction, support, and buy-in is required for growth to occur. Growth here also utilizes a large amount of available resources. Examples of these behaviors might include paying bills, talking with an apartment leasing office, managing an overflowing toilet, problem solving with a professor or manager, or living with a roommate.

63

Breaking down skills into these categories is enormously helpful in devising a plan that can offer an almost mathematical (and personalized) equation for how much stress is healthy and can be handled, and what could be causing damage.

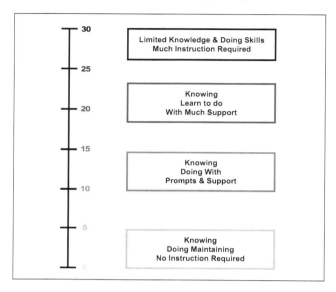

Below in the example of Elizabeth is an illustration of the use of finding balance while taking on challenges.

Elizabeth

Elizabeth was excited for college. For the last five years she had been attending a boarding school with a program designed for students with learning and social disabilities, and she had learned lots through this experience. She was more comfortable around others, was doing well academically, and had developed a good understanding for her own strengths and weaknesses. Elizabeth said she was ready for the next challenge, and everyone working with her agreed. Elizabeth was also ready for the added freedom that would come with life away from a boarding school environment. She had big plans for herself...

However, as with many in her position, this transition turned out to be more than she had anticipated. Elizabeth was now in a totally different environment, and this was surprisingly difficult. No longer in a small town, her primary coping skill of long walks in the country, were no longer available. While a larger city and campus had lots of new and exciting opportunities she wanted to take advantage of, they also tended to be overstimulating. And without a quiet and secluded place to unwind, she struggled to find ways to recharge her internal resources.

Although Elizabeth was doing well in school, her classes and tutoring took up a lot of energy. There were also the added expectations that she remain socially active, that she manage her own budget, and her apartment living skills instructor had expectations for a clean living space and other skill development throughout each semester. This was all very taxing.

For Elizabeth however, the challenges did not end here. She also had a roommate. While Elizabeth had lived with roommates successfully in the past, and this was something she very much wanted, it was also becoming another energy drain. Having a roommate required compromise and communication, and most significantly, required Elibeth to "be on" even while at home. Needing to be respectful of their needs, and to share common space, Elizabeth did not have a place where she could just be herself. Instead, she was engaging in a process of constant self-monitoring, and always felt observed. This alone was very taxing.

Very early into the semester Elizabeth was operating on emergency energy reserves. As a result, she was not coping well. Tearful and distraught one minute, angry the next, Elizabeth was finding it difficult to even leave her apartment each day. She was quickly falling behind, and everyone working with her was enormously concerned. Elizabeth was beating herself up for being a "failure at life and at college." Clearly a change in strategy was required.

In response, Elizabeth, her psychologist and parents reassessed her abilities, and drew up a ranking of those major daily tasks Elizabeth was expected to manage. They were ranked by the level of ease at which they were currently being performed.

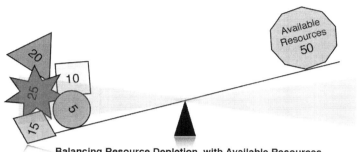

Balancing Resource Depletion, with Available Resources

Identification and use of new emotional coping
     skills within an urban & collage environment 25
Living with a roommate 20
Expectations for social involvement 15
Managing the tasks of independent living 10
Managing current academic expectations 5

                                      75

It was clear the current expectations required a level of energy that exceeded Elizabeth's resources. Something very clearly needed to change.

After much discussion, it was determined moving her into a single apartment was the most logical adjustment to be made. While deeply disappointing to Elizabeth and her parents, this move served two important purposes. First, it reduced Elizabeth's requirement for social interaction. Now, instead of putting her in a situation requiring social discourse and self-regulation during most daylight hours, she had greater control over when these interactions occurred. Secondly, this adjustment also provided a substitute for her previous coping skill of walking in the country. While very clearly not the same, Elizabeth's apartment could become a place of quiet refuge, a reasonable adaptation to city living. Elizabeth could meditate and have quiet time, and she could pursue her individual hobbies without concern of inconveniencing her roommate. In short, Elizabeth's apartment became a place where she could re-charge her energy reserves, rather than a place that did the opposite.

Predictably, this adjustment brought Elizabeth back in balance.

As predicted by the research on self-regulation and resource depletion, Elizabeth's exposure to new and challenging tasks, followed by sufficient rest and re-charging, resulted in an increased ability to manage stress. Thus the psychological weight of many daily tasks decreased with time. This allowed for the introduction of new challenges, including the reintroduction of the roommate experience, expectations for even greater levels of responsibility, a greater number of academic credits per semester, and employment.

These types of adjustments are never ending…

While Elizabeth became increasingly able to monitor and find this balance on her own, she still required occasional coaching from her parents.

Ultimately though, this well-timed feedback made the difference between success and failure for Elizabeth. Resulted in her achievement of great and unexpected things.

Observation Exercise

1. How do you know when your Breakaway's internal reserves of energy are depleted to a level that effects functioning?
2. When levels are depleted what are the typical behaviors you observe? Do they act out, become agitated, withdraw, engage in negative self talk, sleep, etc.?
3. What situations tend to be the most resource-depleting?
4. Is this predictable?
5. What sensory issues are in the environment that might influence energy reserves?
6. Are there seasonal influences?
7. How do diet and sleep influence, or are influences by, resource depletion?
8. What positive coping skill do you observe your young adult using when resources are depleted?
9. Describe situations where you have tried, and found success, in increasing your young adult's resiliency. Why was it a success?
10. Describe situations where you have tried, and did not succeed, in increasing your young adult's resiliency in a stress-inducing situation. What happened to make it unsuccessful?

Notes

Notes

The Breakaway

Identity Development

*A desire to be observed, considered, esteemed, praised,
beloved, and admired by his fellows is one of the earliest
as well as the keenest dispositions discovered
in the heart of man.*

John Adams

The Breakaway

The need to belong is as old as humankind.

Early man came together and formed groups both for companionship and as a means of survival. There was power in numbers, and comfort in knowing one was not facing the darkness of night alone. Within a group, responsibilities could be divided, productivity and creativity increased, and the fortunes of all improved. Staying together was imperative, the consequences of being ostracized, or worse, banished, was literally life-threatening.

Today, it may no longer be life-or-death, but the psychological effect of social isolation over time can prove almost as devastating. The ability to connect with others is still a crucial factor in a person's well-being. Everyone wants to feel safe in the company of a group and to gain their acceptance despite one's flaws and idiosyncrasies. It is that universal need to be admired, to find a place where you fit in, where you can be nurtured and appreciated, that is a huge motivator of an individual's behavior.

For the Breakaways, a positive social identity through group affiliations can sometimes feel near impossible. Labelled by their peers as Special Ed, disabled, autistic, and yes, even "stupid", "creepy", or "weird", they are often singled-out and avoided, or else lumped together with other "loners" only for derision.

They need to feel connected, and to identify with something unrelated to their disability status. Something with a perceived higher social value.

If this does not occur, individual coping skills will continue to decrease over time as this struggle drains their resources. This includes behavioral self-regulation, cognitive flexibility, organization, and decision-making skills. Additionally, long-term rejection has been shown to result in an increased occurrence of depression, eating disorders, anger, aggression, sexual promiscuity, physical pain, suicidal ideation, and self-injurious behavior.

Thus it is critically important that you support your Breakaway as they work to build their identity through group affiliations and external affirmation. ***Be assured that this can and will happen.*** Even if this success is initially found in areas that feel (to you) immature or unusual, these explorations are essential.

Their trial-and-error experiments with different interests, opinions, subcultures and dress are likely to look and feel quite random, even counterproductive to your agenda of helping them feel and act less awkward, or to develop age-appropriate, mainstream or "normal" interests, but this behavior is in fact energizing and critical to the process of identity development.

It's important to note that at any given time we are all affiliated with several distinct groups. Together they comprise the multi-dimensional nature and uniqueness of each individual. A group may be as broad as gender, or as specific as a bowling team or an interest in Anime. Your young adult will determine the value of what their membership in each group means to them, not you. These affiliations will inspire different levels of closeness, and are likely to shuffle around in priority and intensity of interest quite often.

This is an ever-evolving process, where they will work to separate from family and seek out connections where they feel accepted and new activities with peers who they admire.

It is a period of reinvention and role-playing similar to what neurotypical kids go through at ages 12, 13, or 14. The difference, of course, is the stakes can be much higher at this later age. Classes, meetings, and jobs must be attended. Too much time rebelling, testing limits, or "finding one's self" can result in further setbacks and disappointment.

Eventually though it should lead to a more positive reframing of their diagnosis – *"Yes I'm a Aspie, and I love it!"*, or, *"I'm an Aspie and it isn't the end of the world"* - and efforts to make this status more appealing to others - *"Aspie's may be socially awkward, but they drive all the innovation in the tech industry..."*, *"You know, (talented musician) is an Aspie"*.

This reframing of status for self and others is especially important, as it is not healthy to ever entirely disavow the group affiliation associated with their diagnosis.

At a time in life when it seems possible, maybe for the very first time, to redefine who one is and what one might become, a willful denial of their diagnosis can give them a false sense of being "cured". A complete rejection and avoidance of anything associated with the ASD community will only magnify, not conceal, their disability.

To illustrate this point, let us consider the following case study.

Jeff

For Jeff, who did not have his learning difference, and 2e status, identified, until his freshman year of college, the idea of acknowledging his "diagnosis" or seeking assistance was impossible to imagine. He wanted no part of it. It was a label, and he did not subscribe to the idea that anyone should be judged or labeled. Especially b y the psychiatric and educational communities! Instead, Jeff planned to charge ahead in much the same manner as he always had.

Besides, this approach had been proven to be successful...

Although a little awkward growing up, Jeff had found some success with peers. Despite his undiagnosed learning difference, Jeff was actually quite skilled at adapting his social style to mirror the behavior of peers or adults. He was good at blending in, and skilled in hiding what he did not know or understand. He looked to others for information about how to dress and behave, by just following their lead. While at times uncomfortable, this approach was very effective at hiding most of his deficits from others.

Upon reflection, his parents described Jeff as a social chameleon. His interests and style changed to reflect whomever he was with. Consequently, it was never easy to get a sense of who Jeff was or how he felt about things. Their son generally agreed with the ideas of others and did little to draw attention to himself.

Adults liked Jeff and most peers found him funny. Jeff however found the most success socially with peers experimenting with alcohol and drugs. It was within this group that his deficits were even less obvious and he felt a sense of coolness that he did not experience in other areas of his life. Because his behavior with adults was typically appropriate and charming, this area of Jeff's life was never identified, and thus never became an acknowledged problem despite his pattern of abuse.

Academically Jeff's grades were adequate. Not great, but acceptable enough not to be flagged as an area of great concern. Despite his deficits, Jeff had average cognitive abilities and had successfully utilized a combination of cheating and charming teachers to compensate for his slow processing speed, difficulties composing his thoughts, and poor organization skills. He graduated high school with a 2.8 grade point average, and from all accounts was expected to manage well on his own in college.

He was attending the same university his parents had attended and relished the attention he was receiving from family and friends for the accomplishment of his admission and his new identity as a college student. He was proud of himself.

However, once there, Jeff's established coping skills did not find as much success in this new environment. He could establish superficial friendships but struggled to develop meaningful relationships with others. Friends tended to come and go and he became more isolated as he worked to conceal areas of weakness. He struggled to fit in with peers in the same way he had in high school, as academic focus and achievement were increasingly important. This was an area of weakness for Jeff and it was one that was becoming difficult to hide.

With less structure than ever before Jeff had found it difficult to make it to class on time, or at all, and was struggling to keep up with the work load. Professors were immune to his charm, he found it difficult to cheat, and he was afraid to let anyone know he needed help. Jeff's grades were poor and getting worse. He was quickly on academic probation and at risk for dismissal from the university.

In response to these obvious difficulties, Jeff's parents stepped in. They enlisted the help of a local psychologist who provided and confirmed the presence of his previously identified learning difference, as well as a diagnosis of Major Depression - Mild. Suggestions for next steps were made, including the utilization of resources at the campus Student Access Center, extra tutoring, medication, and supportive counseling. While all of this was helpful, it was also extremely jarring.

Nothing about this diagnosis was consistent with who Jeff had always been told he was, nor who he *wanted* to be. He preferred being the clever underachiever to being an individual with disabilities; someone with labels, someone less socially desirable. Jeff was very worried if this information got out others would see him as stupid, or even "retarded". In no way was this acceptable. He would rather continue playing the role of everyone's favorite slacker. Anyway, he could do better if he wanted – he wasn't going to be told what to do!

Jeff was conflicted. Deep down he knew he needed help, but would only accept it on his own terms and his own timeframe. He managed to convince his parents (who also wanted to see Jeff as "normal") to not follow the recommendations of the psychologist for an extended "trial period". He got them to buy into the idea that it was harmful to his psyche to be seen in a tutor center where there might be peers with more obvious or self-identified disabilities, that he could cope without medication or counseling, and that measured marijuana use was the most effective treatment for managing anxiety or winding down at the end of a hard day.

The entire family shared in his denial.

Jeff was sharp, facile and capable of achieving. But he was also experiencing a crisis of identity – whole-heartedly committed to an increasingly obvious and ineffective lie.

Finally, after a period of struggle and profound back-sliding, Jeff gave in and accepted the assistance available to him.

For their part, his parents also made peace with the reality of Jeff's obstacles, and Jeff himself. They needed time to absorb his diagnosis and realize it was okay.

With the help of their psychologist they all became closer, and as a family were able to construct a new identity for Jeff that acknowledged his areas of weakness without emphasizing them. They helped him to see that many highly successful and famous individuals had faced similar challenges, and there was no shame in advocating for the support he needed on the path to his own success.

In short, they helped Jeff to dream again.

The Dilemma of Disability

Many developing young adults with ASD, or 2e are confronted with this same dilemma. They refuse to discuss deficits, and will not accept assistance for fear of being "outed".

This only limits their positive interactions with others, and the recognition of their unique strengths, as all energy is sapped by the unnecessary concealment of deficits.

However, for Breakaways struggling to formulate an identity, convinced others are watching their every move, such self-awareness does not come easy. It may take many ups and downs before they come to a true understanding of themselves

While this is happening, a parent's role does not change.

Without question, the behavior you observe might be frustrating, but it does serve a purpose. Your Breakaway may not be taking the most direct route to their destination, or in a way that makes sense to you, but they are learning the lessons needed to get there. They are just doing it at their own pace, with the tools they possess. They are trying on different identities like clothes in front of a mirror; searching for one that fits, a flattering reflection, and vitally, one that will be approved by others. Group identification plays a huge role.

The Maturity Gap

Most discussions I have with parents deal with their concerns about delayed social skills and interests. By this age, parents are impatient for their child to grow up. As a result, some may discourage an interest in books, music, activities, and even friends that do not feel "mature" enough. But the desire to engage with the world, define oneself and discover one's personal tastes, is a net positive no matter how juvenile it may seem.

Here are a few examples…

Leslie

Leslie, an outgoing and eager 18 year-old was excited to take classes at the local community college. While it was still unclear if she would be able to overcome her learning disabilities to complete an associate's degree, the remedial classes she was taking, provided a great opportunity for her to mature and see what she could do on her own. Leslie's parents were also eager to see her have a college experience. They remembered with great fondness the friendships and adventures they had in college, and wanted the same for their daughter. To their surprise (and frustration), Leslie did not show a similar interest in these college behaviors.

Instead, Leslie chose to maintain the friendships she had developed in high school with younger peers. She continued to show great interest in pre-teen/tween program-ming of the Disney Channel and Nickelodeon. She never missed her favorite shows, frequented fan websites, and followed the music that many of the shows promoted. Her walls were covered with posters of her favorite male stars, and she would often spend afternoons with friends drawing in coloring books and gossiping incessantly about peers and celebrities. Conflicts, disagreements, and "drama" with friends took up most of her time. This was definitely not "college-age" behavior, and was not consistent with the significant transition that she had made.

Out of frustration, Leslie's parents restricted her television viewing, discouraged contact with existing peers, and signed her up for a volunteer organization on campus. They were hoping that this would help her develop more age appropriate friends and interests. Unfortunately, this approach only seemed to make Leslie hold tighter to her familiar, and less mature, interests and behaviors.

Tim

Like Leslie, Tim was transitioning to life after high school. He was taking community college classes, and was also exploring areas of interest that required more of a trade school education. Tim however was more focused on being perceived as grown-up, as being "cool," and as someone that would not be picked on by others. He wanted to be accepted, and to have a girlfriend. Most importantly, he did not want to be anything like his parents!

To reach these goals Tim decided to become a rock-star. He began to wear rock-star jewelry, cloths reminiscent of the 80's hair bands, and carried drumsticks everywhere he went - even class. Tim wanted to form a band and become a star. If that did not pan out, his second choice was to channel his musical talents into a career as a music producer. This is what was most important to him. School was a distraction to his main interest, but he was willing to attend if it meant continued financial support from his parents.

This drove Tim's parents crazy. From their perspective Tim had no real talent for music, and they did not have the resources to let him play at being a rock-star. It was time for him to learn the skills he would need to support himself. They did not want to support him forever, and were anxious about his lack of urgency or ambition to get on with his life. This led to frequent arguments. They were critical of the way he dressed, the friends he was choosing, and his lack of interest in school. For his part, Tim became increasingly rebellious, and did not feel understood or supported by his parents.

Jack

Jack loved everything about the Civil War, and longed to be a historical reenactor. His bookshelf was full of books on the subject, he played battle games, and wore a Union cap on a daily basis. While he could easily have conversations on other topics, he was not interested. This was his passion and main area of interest.

To everyone's frustration, Jack seemed uninterested in considering other topics, even if they were part of a specific course curriculum. To his credit, Jack was taking a full load of college classes and maintaining an acceptable GPA - with much required redirection. So while he had a very restricted range of interest, he was progressing through his classes, and not rebelling against the support he needed.

Jack's parent's had noticed that his focus on the Civil War increased with his stress level, and did wonder if this behavior was serving a purpose as a coping skill. If this was the case, they were hesitant to push for changes. However, they were quite concerned that his restricted range of interest would limit his ability to make friends, and to find future employment. After all, what employer would let Jack wear his hat to work every day...? It would be nice if Jack could incorporate his interest in the Civil War into an overall identity that included more than one dimension. Was that too much to expect from someone with ASD? They didn't know what to do.

Most parents confronted with such circumstances would struggle with how to respond. It is true that if unchanged some of these behaviors might well limit their kids' future opportunity, but unrealistic expectations and condemnation of the behaviors doesn't seem reasonable either. A larger perspective is needed before jumping in with a response.

For Leslie, Tim, and Jack, their seemingly stunted or regressive actions were serving a purpose. *Along with the bonus of frustrating and puzzling their parents, these behaviors were providing a sense of identity, belonging, and connection.*

Leslie was clinging to familiar interests, and to those relationships where she knew the rules and felt appreciated for who she was. While this had yet to happen in the "real world" of adulthood, Leslie knew she would always be accepted by her younger set of friends. They provided a comfort zone, a safe foundation from which she could push herself to face new challenges and develop new skills.

To this end, gossip and drama with friends was also functional. The re-telling of their own and other's social missteps was reinforcing and instructive. Through gossip they were correcting one another's behavior, and learning a new set of rules needed to live up to more adult social expectations. *Taking this away from her would not be a constructive approach in promoting her growth and maturity.*

Unlike Leslie, Jack had found an interest (the Civil War) that might develop into something bigger. It could be a career, and it was an area of interest valued by other adults. He was, however, not currently interested in exploring future options, or even discussing topics that did not directly relate to his interest. He was over-identifying with this subject at the expense of exploring other avenues, or expanding his level of knowledge. Jack was, however, learning to function in the world and making real strides. He, too, had found a comfort zone. ***Its removal, or any devaluing of this interest by those providing support, would be a big mistake.***

For his part, Tim was actively engaging in a process of role-playing. Reminiscent of behaviors observed in a thirteen year-old, he was rebelliously trying on different personas that he had observed on television, in the movies, on social media – in this case, the Rock star – in order to be "special" deliberately, stand out and provoke a reaction. With limited to no actual talent, this pursuit may seem a waste of time, but it still serves the very real purpose of allowing him to exercise his freedom and grow his self-esteem. He was maturing, progressing through a stage of development common to everyone's experience, just a little bit later than usual. ***The challenge for his parents is to grit their teeth and allow this development to run its full course, without compromising his ability to meet real-world expectations for someone his age.***

In all three case, the parents must resist the impulse to restrict these interests, but instead, encourage a balance and expansion of interests whenever possible.

Just like the parents mentioned above, your challenge is to try and understand such quirky behavior in its proper context. This need to identify with and feel connected with others will quite often come before their need to meet your expectations. They will continue to need your support, as they work to establish an identity and acceptance from others, which will allow them to be both part-of and separate from family.

Remember: not all poor decisions or adverse experiences result in life-altering and negative consequences. Exploration of one's likes and obsessions, identification with other groups and individuals, are all a net positive, even if they ultimately turn out to be a poor fit. Disappointment, detours, and setbacks are all part of the process. They will, however, benefit from your continued guidance as you help them to recognize there are other more socially rewarding groups they could and do belong to because of their talents and interests.

One must not forget that along with the challenges faced as a part of ASD, or 2e, these Breakaways are also facing the same developmental hurdles as their peers. Their timing may not be the same, but the trials and tests they face and their need to manage them with success, are very much the same.

Identity Development Questions

1. What groups have you seen your Breakaway wanting to associate with?

2. In what group or groups do you see them most easily finding acceptance?

3. What group affiliations have you seen your young adult wanting to avoid?

4. Do the affiliations your Breakaway is hoping to establish meet your approval?

5. How has your developing young adult responded to social isolation and ostracism?

6. How comfortable are you in discussing with your young adult their diagnosis and disabilities?

7. How well do they understand their diagnosis and the obstacles they present on a daily basis?

8. What level of awareness does your young adult have about their need for support and coaching?

9. Is your young adult aware of their need for support and coaching?

Notes

Accountability

A new position of responsibility will usually show a man to be a far stronger creature than was supposed.

William James

The Breakaway

Have you ever seen someone start out with great plans for achievement only to fail to finish or, worse yet, fail to even start? Whether out of fear of failure, limited organizational skills, or an inability to shift from a dreaming mode to one of action, just getting started can be difficult. The best intentions and even the most well-articulated plans are not enough; another very significant element is needed.

That element is *Accountability*.

Webster's defines Accountability as a state of being answerable to others for one's actions and efforts. It is essential to individual performance and persistence, and most of all, a sense of ownership. In fact, this is why most effective weight-loss, twelve-step and fitness programs all incorporate a group component. The supportive accountability that comes through such "team" relationships refines one's efforts in a positive direction. Knowing that others are watching instills in any person a greater sense of purpose and responsibility. Not surprisingly, ambition increases and more is achieved.

Accountability is about establishing external pressures that highlight the benefits of change. Remember, the discomfort they experience by not changing needs to outweigh the discomfort experienced when learning to do things differently. Accountability is that tipping point.

Every year I come across students (and their parents) who are not ready to face the shift in expectations that occurs when leaving the relative protection of high school. Many have become accustomed to receiving an accommodation or modification for anything difficult, with others problem-solving for them or jumping in to smooth the way; thus they have little to no awareness of their existing skill set. The unfortunate result is a young adult with limited self-determination, and quite often, a misplaced sense of entitlement.

The simple fact is your Breakaway will probably have to work harder than others. They must come to accept this. They must learn to make the active decision to do that extra work. To do it for their present and their future. The burden has shifted from you and other caretakers onto their own shoulders. Even when situations seem unfair or are unfair, they need to face and manage those setbacks with intention rather than passivity, in a more strategic well-thought-out manner. *Any perpetuation of victimhood has to be discouraged at all costs.*

This may sound harsh, I know – but it's important to remember that, in general, the world at large does not care about (or change for) anyone's deficit or disability. Most of the time, people just don't want to be inconvenienced by them. What does matter, however, especially to potential educators and employers, is an attitude of determination and genuine effort to do the best of one's ability. That's an attitude people can work with!

Inappropriate and non-age appropriate behavior will not be forgiven like it might have been during earlier stages of development. For example, poor hygiene, missed deadlines, rude comments or disruptive tangents will not be acceptable in these new environments. Breakaways will be expected to use good judgment, to focus, to self-adjust, to finish what they start, and to accept the consequences of their actions. The world will expect them to possess these skills and more – or will replace them with those who do.

Yes, most people will make reasonable accommodations for difference or disability, but a strong work ethic and reliability always come first.

Your challenge is to make sure they are ready to face these grown-up expectations by keeping them accountable and *not displacing their responsibility*.

Avoiding the 80/20 Trap

Like most behaviors, the displacement of responsibility is learned.

In earlier stages of development, many parents have modeled a pattern of frustration with schools, tutors, administrators and support providers at the first sign of trouble in their child's progress. This sometimes subtle, sometimes less-than-subtle, shifting of responsibility onto professionals for "allowing" the child to experience discomfort, or "failing to do enough" to help the child, inadvertently teaches displacement and blame. While this might feel appropriate and satisfying in the moment, it sends the wrong message; and by the time kids reach young adulthood it can stunt their progress, as they feel no true ownership of their skill-level.

For parents striving to facilitate a smooth transition, this can establish a disastrous pattern we call the *The 80/20 Trap*. This is where the parents are still handling decisions, chores and even emotions that should no longer be their domain. They continue to be responsible for 80% of the results achieved, while their (would-be) Breakaway simply follows, or is pulled along. Stalled, with only 20% control of their own life. Still in that passenger seat.

This very clearly does not represent a path toward personal ownership, or a sense of confidence, in one's efforts. Aspiring young adults are robbed of the opportunity to see what they can accomplish through their own hard work. It will also lead to guaranteed failure whenever the parent finally steps away.

What we are seeking is for those percentages to be reversed: *with the young person providing 80% of the effort, and the support team providing the assisting 20% as needed.*

As a rule, accommodations should be made only to support *existing skills*, not to compensate for poor effort, or provide excuses *for skills that should have been developed by now, but still have not been fully grasped and mastered.*

Below are two case studies that illustrate common mistakes that are made when wrestling with this issue of accountability...

Denise

By mid-semester Denise had a 75% average in her math class. While she could have done better, given her history of struggles in math, she was satisfied to be passing the course. Denise was especially glad to share this news with her father the following week during their Father/daughter ski vacation which dad had set up at the beginning of the semester. However, when she told her math professor she would be missing class the following week, he reminded her she had already used her eight allotted absences for the semester, and that each additional absence would result in a letter-grade drop at the class's completion.

Upon hearing this news, Denise's father was incensed. Instead of holding Denise accountable, he immediately called her professor, followed by her academic advisor, and finally the department Dean. He yelled and screamed, claiming that Denise's diagnosis made it difficult to sustain the same level of effort as other students, that she was especially fragile, that she needed a break, and finally that he only had limited time during the year for these visits. To the frustration of her professor and those teaching her the skills of personal responsibility and accountability to others, he ultimately was able to obtain a special exception for his daughter. At no time did he question Denise, or hold her accountable for the absences she had accumulated, which was ultimately a lost learning opportunity for her.

Cooper

Through a connection with family friends, Cooper was able to get a job filing and answering the phone at a local business. Although this was his first job, Cooper's parents assured the office manager that he was more than capable of taking on the duties listed in the job description. However, after three weeks on the job Cooper was fired because this was not the case. As it turned out, Cooper struggled in multiple areas; this included his difficulty to consistently file charts in alphabetical order, tardiness to work, a resistance to following directions, and a desire to do things his own way and at his own pace. Cooper also frequently smelled as if he had not bathed, making him difficult to be around.

Cooper's mom was sad to hear the news. She immediately went to the employer's office and spoke to the manager. During this meeting she demanded that Cooper be given a second chance, and that maybe his job responsibilities could be reduced to fit his current skill set. After all it was just his first job, and he did have Autism. The office manager responded by saying they had already spent an excessive number of hours on training Cooper, that they had been very clear about the job duties before he was hired, and they could not afford to have an employee who could not perform all of the required tasks. When the office manager suggested it might be a good idea to contact the local Vocational Rehabilitation Center to tap into their job training programs, her anger increased and she threatened to sue. She would find him another job, with a more understanding and less discriminatory employer.

In subsequent conversations with Cooper, she focused on her feelings about the employer, the discrimination he had experienced, and where she would find him his next job. At no time did they discuss the nature of his current skills, or Cooper's role in failing to meet the job requirements

Just as with Denise, this too was a missed opportunity for a valuable learning experience. Unfortunate.

If this pattern sounds familiar, if you find yourself more focused on preventing discomfort and setbacks, rather that expecting personal responsibility, it is not too late to shift to a more productive path: an approach that presumes any individual seeking independence must be a full participant in the daily decisions that affect their life. Encourage them to make choices, let them make mistakes, hold them accountable, and assist them as they regroup and repeat the cycle, learning to do so with greater and greater independence.

Unfortunately, there is no shortcut here. The development of these skills will take much practice, many stumbles, and much reinforcement from you.

Living in the world with any type of disability or deficit is hard. Some amount of sadness, anger and grief about this reality is appropriate. However, one cannot get stuck there. The definition of adulthood is pushing through, moving on. Failure should never be casually written off as the result of a difficult teacher or boss, personality conflicts, bigotry, a lack of accommodation, etc. This is what the world throws at them and it is what they will have to deal with for the remainder of their lives.

Obviously, you will continue to contribute emotional and financial support, coaching, tutoring, etc., celebrating each small victory and encouraging gains in maturity regardless of the immediate outcome. There is no shame in staying attentive and fully engaged. Just make sure your praise is linked to hard work and real growth, not any one single result.

Someone is always watching, seeing their effort and rooting them on.

As long as they know that, even as they are weaned off your direct intervention, you can reverse the 80/20 trap and set the path for great achievement.

Supporting Without Doing

As I said before, we all need others to support our efforts. However, it doesn't help in the long run if they continually do what is difficult for us, thereby robbing us of that experience and the skills to fend for ourselves when they are no longer around.

It is important to clarify – when we discuss accountability, we are not referring to punishment, just the 'normal' social compact where a goal is agreed upon and the individual in question is expected to do their part to make it happen: taking initiative, applying their all, advocating for what they need, and meeting their obligations. In a professional arena, this dynamic can best be observed between an office manager and his/her employees. The office's output is dependent on the combined efforts of the entire personnel, with each worker knowing and fulfilling their own well-defined role.

The manager has created *a culture of accountability* that keeps it all running smoothly. In turn, that culture has been internalized by each employee.

In the case of a transitioning college student, parents may take responsibility for providing alarm clocks, a day-planner, even reminder calls to support the need to be on-time. However, punctuality, as a trait, is unlikely to appear with regularity if it is never internalized sufficiently enough to occur away from the parent's watchful eye.

For a trait to "stick", it has to be understood and felt at a gut level, not enforced.

And it stands to reason if someone is to be measured and evaluated, they need to not only know what they are being evaluated on, but have input into the formation of the "test" (what we earlier called the "Buy-In"). This is the only way that they can learn to effectively direct their efforts toward meeting or exceeding those expectations. Otherwise they will continue avoiding responsibility whenever possible, easily lose their way in the stress of each day and only increase the stress levels of everyone around them.

Therefore, try to explain to your Breakaway each component of accountability.

What is a Goal?

A Goal is a broad statement of purpose that arises from a specific identified need. For each Goal, you will need to develop a strategic plan.

What is a Strategic Plan?

A Strategic Plan breaks down the Goal into specific behaviors or stages that are designed to be measurable. They bluntly state the intent of what you are planning to do and how you are going to get there. For example, if, as above, punctuality is the goal, being on-time to work and school, then a Strategic Plan breaks down the specific behaviors that must be enacted to meet this goal (setting alarms, programming timer on your phone, leaving home by a specific time, being in bed by 11 pm, etc).

Much like journalism, a Strategic Plan should address five essential questions:

Who?

Who is the responsible person? Who will be held accountable for meeting this objective?

What?

What is the tactic or method for the achievement of each objective? For example: "John will set his alarm each night, to go off by 7 am." Additional steps are then added. The goal can be broken down into many small actions, different steps. Just remember, one step at a time. Combining them is confusing, and difficult to measure.

When?

When do we expect to achieve said goal? When first working to develop a behavior, we want to set easy, lenient timelines that will result in a feeling of success. We are gradually building one skill/step/success on top of another until we have mastered an entire task. For example, we may aim for successfully setting the alarm 3 out of 5 nights, just to get started. At the end of the week, progress is evaluated and the expectation changed accordingly. We start with a low bar and then increase the level of difficulty, giving a sense of real forward moment.

Why?

As their parent and coach, it is your job to be sure that your Breakaway does not lose focus on what they are working toward, The Big Picture. It will be easy for them to get bogged down in aggravation and discouragement. While you will not be able to eliminate these struggles, a jolt of motivation can be found in reminding them of The Overall Goal. This can be accomplished with reminder notes or charts to track progress. Say things like *"Being on time is an essential skill needed for living independently"*, or, *"Going to class every week is challenging, but it will give you the grades you need to get that job and salary you want"*. Keeping up this dialogue is important. Keep their eyes on the prize.

How?

How do they react to this challenge? Are they willing and eager to be held accountable? If not, then step back and remind them of their own ambitions, their previous Buy-In. For them to succeed, they absolutely must embrace the idea of being accountable. They must be willing to accept and follow your guidance. If not, slow down, start over, and be sure it catches their enthusiasm this time. Once again, you have to meet them where they are, not where you want them to be.

A culture of accountability does not mean that you are always right, or that your list of priorities and theirs are always the same. It is an ongoing conversation about goals and steps that, hopefully, arise organically out of the Breakaway's wants and needs. Sometimes they will concentrate their energy in an area that seems like an unnecessary detour to you, but go along with it, so A) they see your new equality/collaboration is for real, B) you value their priorities, and C) they get another opportunity to gain confidence. ***Their own self-activated creativity should never be marginalized.*** For individuals all too often defined by what they can't do, the internal rewards that come from their developing sense of autonomy are invaluable. Your patience will be critical here while you build trust.

The story of Grant provides a great example of this delicate dance…

Grant

Convinced that he was destined to be the next internet entrepreneurial million-aire, Grant had no interest in taking college classes. Instead, he preferred to concen-trate on the development of his web-based business in the comfort of his own apart-ment - while continuing to be fully supported by his parents.

To their credit, his parents saw great promise in their son, and his idea of an internet-based business. They were, though, also aware that at age 18, Grant did not yet possess the maturity, knowledge, experience, and financial stability to find the immediate success he was convinced was just within his reach. To them, a college environment, and college classes, were a way for him to find this much needed growth and maturity. Instead of a full-time focus on business development, they proposed that Grant continue to rely on their financial support, while supporting his business with relevant course work. As they told him, "take our money, build your business, and pass some classes". Grant however wanted none of it, and dug in for a long power struggle.

Rather than engaging in a protracted fight, Grant's parents worked to achieve some level of Buy-In. They agreed to let him pursue his business plans full-time, but also reduced their financial support to the very basics - room and board. Grant was now on a very tight budget, and dependent upon the revenue he generated to cover many of his expenses.

While in many ways this felt like a significant detour from their ultimate goal of independence and maturity, Grant's parents did not lose sight of the long-term ob-jective. In order to maintain some level of Buy-In, they simply reworked the strategy to accommodate Grant's current need for autonomy. And they were soon rewarded for their flexibility. After six months of both success and struggles, Grant developed a level of self-knowledge needed to move away from his rigid stance of complete autonomy. He learned he did not know everything he needed to know, that clients do not always pay their bills, that it is hard work developing a business, and that he needed to improve his people skills to achieve HIS ultimate goal.

This lead to his decision to take his parents up on their original offer. Take classes and their financial support, while also continuing to build and refine his business.

While it is easy to see the effectiveness in this approach after the fact, it is important to note it was not easy or automatic. Most parents find it difficult to let go of the most obvious and direct approach, to take what their developing young adult was willing to give and run with it. In this case, total compliance to the plan of taking classes was a non-starter for Grant. Nothing but endless power struggles and a lack of Buy-In would have resulted from pushing this agenda. Another option needed to be found.

However, the initial steps of moving away from a direct approach did not feel logical at the time, and only increased their feelings of doubt, anxiety, frustration, and outright anger. To their credit, Grant's parents did not direct these feelings toward him for very long, recognizing that forward momentum was critical to the team effort they were trying to nurture. To get there, they were willing to be unconventional in their approach, while facing their own discomfort. Along the way, they also provided an important opportunity for Grant to find ownership in the decisions that were shaping his own life. He may have taken a detour, but he was growing and learning. ***Sometimes two or three steps backwards, or even sideways, is the best strategy for moving forward.***

In fact, Grant's parents had planned for just this contingency. They knew the importance of both his Buy-In and the need for accountability. Prior to being faced with this decision, they had come to understand that such a decision did not constitute "giving in", as long as it made sense within the overall plan, and the uniqueness of Grant. They had already spent a significant amount of time planning this transition with Grant, his psychologist, and high school teachers. They were well-prepared, and felt comfortable in their roles of parent, guide and coach. They felt in control - or at least in as much control as a parent or coach can ever be...

For parents entering this transition with a Breakaway already in the Preparation & Action Stages of Change, who is realistic about their future and less resistant to guidance, your approach is likely to be quite different.

They, too, need structure, but they will be much more willing to accept help and take a more measured route toward their goals.

Brooke

Brooke is a great example of a developing young adult transitioning from the Preparation to Action stage of Change. She knew without doubt that she was destined to become a writer. Since middle school she had loved to spend her time creating stories, narratives and writing down observations into her journal. In high school she had received praise from her teachers, and had even been acknowledged in several writing competitions. In addition to writing for fun, Brooke had also found an opportunity to write movie and video game reviews for a website. She was experiencing much success, and clamoring for more.

To her credit, Brooke was also aware that she had much more learning to do, if she was ever to find her way in the very competitive world of writing. She saw her college classes and the relationships she hoped to develop with professors and peers to be very important in the achievement of her long-term goals.

For that reason, Brooke was eager to accept the tutoring and emotional support she needed to find this success. She actively worked with everyone available to provide support in the development of realistic goals, and more short-term strategies for their achievement. While college did not progress without the expected struggles and setbacks, both she and her support team continued to refer to and modify the strategic plan they had in place. Today, Brooke is close to graduation, and contemplating her next move.

Brooke's readiness and thus approach to this transition was very different from Grant's. It is not better, just different, and full of its own challenges. In contrast to Grant's parents, Brooke's struggled to keep up. They were ready for some major rebellion, resistance etc., and were not ready for the speed with which Brooke needed them to step back. Her parents had planned to have a prominent role in her daily decisions, and subsequently felt lost when Brooke was not interested in them filling that role. They were very uncomfortable. Like Grant's parents, when this occurred, they greatly benefitted from a review of the Strategic Planning that they had done prior to the onset of this transition. This enabled them to step away from the emotion of the moment, to review established long-term goals, and to modify the plans they had developed. Like Grant, Brooke needed to have a clear structure for accountability, and she needed some say in the type/level of support she needed.

Again, I want to stress that accountability is not about punishment or some kind of autocratic control. It is only about the healthy process of shifting responsibility, bit by bit, from the parent to the young adult, for their own safety and protection – and future fulfillment! As difficult as this may feel at times, it is a critical step that must be taken.

All self-determination is dependent on holding oneself accountable.

It's about modeling those skills that will eventually lead your Breakaway to success and the achievement of great things. Sometimes, even, to what right now may seem impossible.

It will not be easy. Both you and your young adult are going to experience a steep learning curve. Maintain a clear line of communication and be as consistent as possible. This consistency will eliminate confusion and mixed messages. It will also help compensate for the many errors that will inevitably be made along the way.

It's your response to those mistakes and lapses that will be key, and require the most judicious and delicate of constructive criticism.

Final Questions

1. How successful have you been at establishing a system of consistent accountability?
2. In what circumstances do you find yourself in the 80/20 Trap?
3. In what circumstances have you observed your Breakaway deflecting responsibility?
4. In what circumstances to you observe your Breakaway taking responsibility for their choices and behavior? How do these circumstances differ from those where they deflect responsibility?
5. In what circumstances do you find it difficult to hold your Breakaway accountable, and to struggle, as a result of their choices they have made?
6. In what circumstances do you find it most easy to hold them accountable?
7. Do you and your spouse/partner agree on when and how to establish a system for accountability? In what areas do you agree? In what areas do you disagree?
8. Think of a situation when the feedback you provided was well received and when it was not well received. What contributed to the outcome of each situation?
9. What was your most important takeaway from this chapter?

Notes

Notes

Feedback

In the absence of effective feedback, people will fill in the blanks with a negative. They will assume you don't care about them or don't like them.

Pat Summitt

The Breakaway

Feedback works hand-in-hand with accountability.

In fact, accountability would be ineffective, and arguably inappropriate, without the direction that effective feedback provides. Presented through verbal and nonverbal forms of communication, the intention of feedback is to motivate, to provide information, and to facilitate development.

Feedback is also a wonderful tool for lowering stress. This occurs through the reduction of uncertainty, as one clarifies what has been done well, what areas need improvement, and what should be done next. This type of communication spells out very clearly what behaviors will grow into further successes and which ones will not. This information is critically important to a population that does not always understand why one situation went well, while a different but very similar situation did not. This is stressful! And as we have discussed when looking at resource depletion and resilience, increased stress results in a decreased ability to process and integrate information. Functioning levels then decrease. By explaining what was done well and what areas need improvement, Breakaways are better able to take that information in and use it to facilitate growth going forward.

Whether providing or receiving, intended or not, feedback is a natural component of our interactions with others. Directly through verbal means, or nonverbally through behavior and facial expressions, one's thoughts, feelings, concerns, or preferences are continually broadcast to those around us. These signals is unavoidable. Even the avoidance of providing feedback itself sends a very clear message to the world.

But does this population of developing young adults really hear what we are saying? Can they really process all of this information? Do we *want* them to receive the message that is being sent? Is the feedback provided in these messages appropriate and effective? Are those on the receiving end open to this feedback? Will they even consider it? All very good questions, posed by many parents with whom I work.

While the answers to each will differ depending on unique circumstances, it is safe to assume that one is sending messages that are being received. For this reason, it is important to be sure they are the ones you are *intending to send*. An awareness for how, when, and why you are providing feedback will not only help you feel more in control, but it will also improve the development of greater accountability.

Your goal as a parent is to maximize the occurrence of desired behaviors while minimizing those behaviors you would like to eliminate. Learning to provide feedback with clear intention, purpose, and good timing is essential. If you can master these techniques, your developing young adult will feel more capable and confident in their abilities, more willing to take on new challenges. But, conversely, if feedback is poorly delivered or ill-timed, they will become more discouraged and less communicative, less manageable.

This chapter will teach you all the different types of feedback, their usefulness, and those situations where they are best applied, so you can provide this valuable information in a manner that is truly helpful and effective.

In short, how to send the right message.

Avoiding Destructive Feedback

Most individuals providing ineffective feedback do so with the best of intentions, typically based in a desire for rapid improvement, greater productivity.

The problem is their delivery, timing or approach is often way off.

Timing may be the most common mistake of all. Challenges faced during this transition period come fast and hard, and it is difficult to navigate them, let alone keep one step ahead. Frustration and impatience are natural reactions to what feels like chaotic change, but as we all know, are not a good place from which to dispense – ***or to hear*** – feedback. Much of the time we have a gut instinct for when any form of (even mild) criticism will only exacerbate a situation. ***Listen to that intuition.*** Take that important moment to consider if you should save that feedback for later when it will be received with some equanimity.

Let's face it, being on the receiving end of destructive feedback is not pleasant for anyone. Feeling attacked, bullied, picked-on or put-down hurts, and can result in wounds that are slow to heal and prove extremely damaging to trust and future collaboration. This is a circumstance you must avoid at all costs.

Here are some common-sense rules for effective feedback that should guide your efforts and shape the manner in which you engage with your young adult.

Be Timely

Timing is important in another way as well. While not wanting to rush and aggravate a volatile situation, it is equally crucial not to let too much time pass either. Feedback is most effective when provided as close as possible to the behavior, situation, or event being evaluated. The more time that passes, as the event or action in question becomes only a memory, the less effective the feedback will become. And the less chance it will be absorbed as a lesson and yield positive change.

Be Specific

Feedback in the form of generalizations or broad brush strokes will not be helpful. Base your feedback on concrete observable behavior or materials. The person receiving feedback should receive sufficient information to pinpoint those specific behaviors that you are wanting to reoccur, or that need further refinement. Again, be very specific.

Be Descriptive, Not Labeling

Describe what you see. There is no need to infer motivation, feelings or intent. These only serve to cloud the issue. Provide examples of behaviors observed, and link them to outcomes that occurred.

Be Vigilant

If one is going to be providing feedback, they had better be attentive to the behavior they are evaluating. There is nothing more bothersome or hurtful than to receive feedback from someone who has clearly not been paying attention. Don't do this...

Be Direct

Say what you mean. It does no good to avoid or to be unclear. Use simple language and get to the point.

Be Realistic

Feedback should be directed toward those behaviors that your developing young adult can currently act upon. While it is easy to overreach and focus on more advanced skills or future goals, stay in the present. Don't make suggestions that are outside the scope of what they can do right now.

Be Sure to Review Established Goals and Strategic Plans

Don't get ahead of yourself. Discuss broader goals, but reinforce efforts toward their achievement by providing feedback on those important, and sometimes tedious, steps toward their achievement.

Be Non-Judgmental

Avoid value-laden comments that may come off as shaming. Fact-based comments are best, even when feeling provoked, frustrated or angry.

Be Sure Not to Engage in Comparisons

The comparison of one individual to another will complicate the point you are trying to make. It does nothing in the way of reinforcing desired behavior or building skills. Instead, it breeds resentment.

Be Aware

The process of providing feedback is often emotional for both sides. Be sensitive to your young adult's feelings, and be aware of your own. If you are angry, anxious, or frustrated, the intention of the feedback you provide may get lost in these emotions. Always slow down, and proceed in a manner that will be most effective for you and your developing young adult.

These ten points can fine-tune your approach, but first you need a deeper understanding of feedback itself and the different roles it plays…

In an effort to explain more clearly, I have broken feedback into three categories based on the intention behind the words. These include the intention to *Motivate*; to *Describe* what is currently occurring; and to facilitate the *Formation* of new behavior. Whether Motivational, Descriptive, or Formative/Corrective, the feedback must always be thoughtful, appropriate to the situation, and as ever, consistent with your intentions.

Feedback as Motivation

Typically associated with a cheering section, where praise and encouragement are provided, this type of feedback is not as one-dimensional as you might assume - or the name implies. Motivational feedback can work in both directions: Positive feedback when things are going well, negative feedback when things are not, and even the absence of feedback altogether - *Extinction*, when wanting to "extinguish" a behavior without engaging in a power struggle.

Each approach has its own way of influencing behavior. When applied with purpose and forethought, it is about nudging behavior almost subconsciously in a desired direction.

Examples of these approaches may include:

"You look great today. I can tell that you put a lot of effort into your personal hygiene and appearance. Nice work!" [Positive Feedback]

"I can't help but notice that you are again 30 minutes late to work. Since it is the third time this week, I am afraid I must write you up." [Negative Feedback]

Or, the absence of feedback, through the deliberate removal of reinforcing responses. Or put more simply: the ignoring of an undesired behavior. This is often combined with the praise of desired behavior in the person of focus, or the praise of desired behavior of another person in close proximity (not to be confused with comparison). This type of feedback can be quite effective. [Extinction]

Positive Feedback = Reinforcement

We all love positive feedback. It's encouraging, and provides incentive to continue what we are doing. It needs to be just as specific as negative feedback. To have maximum impact, establish new behaviors or skills, let your developing young adult know exactly what

102

you are praising and hope to see more of in the future.

Remember, the experience of growth and development is frightening and confusing. Next steps are not always obvious in the midst of all that uncertainty. Positive feedback provides the Breakaway with an energy boost, and much-needed clarification of what they are already doing right. It's invaluable.

Negative Feedback = Punishment

Negative feedback is trickier, of course. It can be just as motivating. It can result in a greater focus and a return to the "correct way" of doing things…but not always. No matter how gently applied it can feel like punishment, and as a result must be used with great caution.

Many parents fall into the trap of concentrating on the negative, rather than the hard-won (and often small) growth that is evident. It should come as no surprise this only decreases drive and alienates a special-needs population

The harsh truth is with this population there is often an unlimited supply of behaviors or habits needing refinement or redirection. It can be difficult to avoid the impulse to point them out each time they are observed. Remember, that this type of ad-hominem criticism, no matter how justified in the moment or what the intention, will quickly turn self-defeating. It will likely result in resistance, evasion, even open rebellion.

In an effort to avoid this punishing interaction, while still giving into the impulse to make comments, some parents try to conceal their real intentions. They learn to lead with a compliment, followed by a pause, and then a "BUT". More negative feedback follows, and their developing young adult gets wise to the trick, learns to tune it all out or rebel out of sheer frustration. While it is true this approach does recognize things that are going well, it also trains the subject to recoil and become defensive, even when positive feedback is being provided. They are waiting for the stinger at the tail of compliment, the dreaded "BUT".

Corrective feedback is inevitable during this transition. It is an integral part of the learning process. Negative comments, however, should be used with caution and a clear understanding of possible unintended consequences. Again, do not be rash and lash out when exasperated. Stop and reflect. Better to bite your tongue until you can phrase it correctly.

Finally, it is important to find that balance between encouragement and reproach, in order not to stifle exploration of new behaviors. ***Don't nit-pick. Choose your battles.*** Build from a stance of affirmative feedback, with appropriately applied intermittent critiques.

No Feedback = Extinction

Based on the principle of removing the reinforcement (attention) that maintains any behavior or response, Extinction can be a highly effective mechanism for changing conduct.

103

An absence of feedback entirely is a very powerful motivator or tool. Underutilized, this lack of response can, ironically, be more impactful (punitive) than negative Feedback, while not eliciting the defensiveness and hurt feelings. It merely involves ignoring the obvious, in this case the undesired behavior. As such, it deprives the individual presenting these undesired behaviors of any reaction at all, refusing to legitimize the behavior with even a negative interaction.

This approach of "No Feedback" isolates. In the absence of feedback, a dynamic is created where the individual not receiving desired levels of attention begins to alter their strategy in an effort to obtain the attention they want. What occurs next is often called an **Extinction Burst**. This involves a short-term burst in the frequency of the undesired behavior - a behavior that has previously been quite effective in fulfilling their needs, but is now being met with a vacuum of no response. For example:

Kagan

Kagan had always been given money whenever he wanted something. That is, until the transition to young adulthood. It was at this point that his parents developed a very clear budget, and had expectations he stick to it. As you might imagine, Kagan was not at all happy. Instead of willingly complying, he passively agreed. He was not ready for the change his parents were suggesting, and had no intention of complying. Instead of trying to manage his money, his spending habits remained the same. He also continued to ask and beg for money like he had always done - just with greater frequency. He got louder and more dramatic, and did everything he could to make his parents cave in, and go back to the old way of operating.

To their credit, they held firm, and Kagan's Extinction Burst decreased with time. Gradually being replaced with new and more age-appropriate behavior - primarily behaviors motivated by the need to stay within budget and please his parents.

Kagan's behavior is a great example of how individuals respond to Extinction.

Focused on the need for attention (his parent's money here), most will initially continue to do more of what they have been doing (not doing laundry, arguing, begging, poor hygiene etc.). This is part of their change process - of letting go of old and ineffective approaches before developing new skills.

The key point to recognize, however, is that they must REALLY come to know that their old behavior is no longer effective. If Kagan's parents had caved in by giving him more money, they would have reinforced his old behavior and continued the cycle. Instead, by standing strong and not responding to (ignoring) his relentless begging and drama, Kagan was only left with the need to develop a new strategy to get his needs met. And he did.

As he was experimenting with new approaches, Kagan's parents shaped the formation of these new behaviors by providing loads of positive feedback in response to those behaviors/skills they wanted to see him develop.

The ostensible drawback with extinction, of course, is it is not as immediately satisfying for the parent who is feeling frustrated by slow progress. Strategic disengagement can feel very counter-intuitive in the moment. But it is precisely this targeted disengagement that makes it such a powerful intervention. Everyone craves attention, and does not feel good in its absence. It is not necessary to hover over every behavior that is not yet on-track or perfect. Instead, by overly attending to any positive behavior (even if it is barely noticeable), while providing a limited or no response to those behaviors you would like to extinguish, you will be sending a very clear message, while avoiding an uglier clash of wills.

A word of caution about *Unintended Extinction* though. This occurs when one forgets to acknowledge existing positive behavior. Motivation and forward progress is easily lost when not reinforced. This is especially true when behaviors are relatively new, but also pertains to well-established behavior. Everyone wants to be acknowledged for positive efforts. When this does not occur, it is disappointing, and the level of effort put forth in the future may decrease.

Most likely, you have experienced this yourself. Have you ever had an employer fail to acknowledge your hard work? Have you ever had a coworker praised while your longstanding history of outstanding work goes unrecognized? How did you feel? How did you respond? Did it change your behavior going forward? I bet it was hard to consistently put forth 100% effort in the face of no appreciation. One might say, you were motivated to work less.

Don't forget about all those areas that are going well for your Breakaway. While they may no longer involve areas of immediate concern, they should not be ignored. It takes a long time for new behavior to solidify into habits. Reinforcement continues to be needed well beyond that point when these behaviors spontaneously occur with great regularity.

Keep reinforcing!

Finally, be aware that just like other forms of motivational feedback, an extinction approach is not always appropriate. *Never ignore unsafe behavior.* Just as it makes no sense nit-picking at someone who is just beginning to learn a new skill, it makes even less sense to ignore unsafe behavior that could cause real harm. You are still the coach and need to apply your own wisdom for when it may be necessary to draw a line.

105

Feedback as Descriptive Information

As its title suggests, Descriptive Feedback provides objective information about what is occurring. This might include the tracking of class attendance, the number of showers taken per week, grades on exams, skill development toward learning to pay one's bills, preparing meals, or participation in social activities. When providing this type of feedback, one is simply pointing out what is occurring - bringing it to their attention. One is providing the information needed to reinforce achievement or to prompt the subject to make needed corrections.

Descriptive or informational feedback is especially effective once a young adult has discovered the intrinsic value or reward found in taking on and overcoming challenges. In other words, they are engaged in the Preparation, Action, or Maintenance stages of change. If they have not yet found the motivation to tackle the challenges of this transition with independence and conviction, proceed with caution – they will probably not perceive even objective facts as anything but criticism. As always, it is best to take it slow, not overreach.

When using descriptive feedback it is important the individual has a clear understanding of what is being measured and how it will be measured going forward. This information should be part of the strategic plans you have developed for short and long-term goals. If well-designed, descriptive feedback can be tracked by the young adults themselves, without assistance.

Three important components will make this possible:

1) Feedback should relate to clearly established expectations. If the goal is a B in College Algebra, progress toward that goal can be tracked by attendance to tutoring and classes, each graded quiz, homework assignment and test. Be sure your young adult understands the connection between what is being tracked and the overall goal.

2) Feedback should be immediate, or as close to immediate as possible.

3) Visual cues for progress made toward the goal should be provided. This can be a graph, chart, etc. Anything that provides a visual representation of what is occurring. This visual element can be especially helpful. It not only tracks progress made toward the goal, but also provides a clear illustration how each small step of the strategic plan relates to the "big picture" achievement, a connection this population often fails to make.

The value of Descriptive Feedback can be seen in the story of Chad.

Chad

Chad was training to be a Veterinary Assistant. He had successfully completed the course work required for his certification, and had thrived in the structure and specific focus the training program had provided. He was now off to complete his externship hours to be performed in a local vet clinic. He was excited, this was his opportunity to both demonstrate what he had learned and to refine skills within an unpredictable, real-life environment. Two hundred successful clinical hours were required for the completion of his program.

Being the linear and compartmentalized guy he was, Chad had a very clearly established goal and was perfectly willing to follow the expectations of his training program, but with this switch to the more dynamic world of a clinic, he struggled to know what to do. His stress levels were up, he wasn't sure how to act, or even how he was doing. In school, he received feedback after each daily quiz. He missed that structure and the reinforcement it provided. He needed something specific to work toward.

In the absence of that structure, Chad created his own.

For him, *the number of hours* he spent at the clinic would be the measure of his achievement. Unfortunately, this narrow focus came at the expense of skills he was meant to be developing during this training experience.

See, Chad's desired client population was lions and tigers, not dogs and cats, so he saw the vet clinic as something completely disconnected from his target work environment, just an obstacle to his ultimate goal of working in a zoo. Like many young adults with Autism Spectrum Disorder, he failed to recognize that goal achievement involved the completion of multiple small steps; some clearly related to the final destination, others not so clearly related, but enormously valuable opportunities to learn nonetheless.

He also did not experience the clinic as an extension of what he had just learned while in class. Thus the information he had demonstrated on quizzes was not transferring to the new situation. In his mind, it was a separate experience, not linked. While the transfer of learning from one situation to another had always been challenging, in this situation he simply was not trying. He expected to be "taught" in the same manner that he had been in class and became a big indignant when this did not occur.

As charming as Chad could be, this approach did not go over well with his supervisors and colleagues. They were frustrated with Chad's lack of initiative and his inability to retain information from one day to the next.

While Chad was focused on the completion of his hours, those working with him were concerned about his ability to do the job and pass his externship. Things were not going well. There was significant doubt that he could become a Vet Assistant.

After much discussion, what became clear to everyone involved, was that Chad was not being provided the type of feedback he needed to be successful. He needed specific and immediate feedback about his performance on a daily basis. He needed to be reminded how skill development was at least equally as important as the completion of hours. He needed a visual representation of the progress he was making toward the development of those skills needed for the achievement of his ultimate goal of working in a zoo. He needed some descriptive feedback to help him monitor his progress, and assistance in reconnecting with his goals and strategic planning. He also really needed much positive feedback to prevent too much discouragement.

As a result of this new understanding, charts were created to track his progress in the different skill areas needed for the completion of his externship. The end goal was to develop each skill to either "Proficient" or "Above Average" levels.

Every day before starting work, Chad and his job coach reviewed his current skill levels and performance the previous day. They also established expectations for the day to come. At the end of that day's work, they again reviewed his performance, and a score was given to each skill he learned or re-performed that day. And, it made a really big difference! Performance and attitude improved, stress levels decreased.

While there was most certainly much positive feedback and formative coaching, the inclusion of ***this well-designed descriptive feedback*** is ultimately what made the difference for Chad.

As with each type of feedback we are discussing, descriptive feedback will not fit all circumstances, but for the developing young adult ready and eager to take a proactive stance, informational updates and the tracking of progress is most effective.

Feedback as Formative Coaching

At some point it will be important to offer feedback that is not just motivational or simply informative. Instruction is needed. Provided within a context that includes these other forms of feedback, Formative Coaching is both instructional and corrective in nature. It can be used to prepare the Breakaway for upcoming challenges and what could be done better next time. For example, *"Be sure to wear the outfit we discussed and to monitor your eye contact*

108

during your job interview", or, *"Yelling at your supervisor was not an appropriate way to resolve that problem. Let's talk about other ways you could have managed that situation".* When provided in a helpful non-threatening manner it can refine skills and build competence.

Some of you may be wondering: How is Formative Feedback different from Negative Feedback? Or – How does this not become punitive? Good questions.

The answer lies in the intention behind the feedback when it is provided, in its timing, and in the pre-existing structure or culture you have developed for evaluating performance. All three are key for avoiding a punitive approach.

When establishing a culture of open communication and accountability, it is essential to have *a consistent format* when discussing performance. The same location, a regular time, a specific ritual. This type of routine creates a level of friendly predictability for all, and provides a needed structure for what otherwise might be an awkward conversation.

I also suggest a structure of verbal steps, or questions, to be addressed in a certain order. These Who's, What's, and What Next's will provide a clear format, create a sense of objectivity, and are non-punishing yardsticks when situations are full of emotion.

One set is for coaching in preparation for a yet-to-be-mastered set of challenges, the other a formative review of past performance. I have found each to be a simple helpful outline that organically, comfortably invites Feedback and Accountability.

The questions are:

PREPARATORY COACHING

1) What is supposed to happen?
2) What are the steps for making this happen?
3) What cues or tools are available to support your efforts?

POST EVALUATION

1) What was supposed to happen?
2) What actually happened?
4) What have we learned?
3) What should we do next?

Given that the purpose behind Formative Coaching is support, it is also important to avoid providing this type of feedback when feeling irritated or annoyed. When this occurs, the intention is lost, and anything constructive will go to waste. The other thing to remember here is the importance in timing one's positive feedback so that it does not get tied to the corrective feedback you provide. *In general, try not to mix too much positive feedback in with your formative coaching*. Confused? Once again, this may seem like contradictory advice, but as we discussed in the Negative Feedback section, leading with a positive comment followed by a negative or corrective statement, trains those on the receiving end to become wary of praise. They come to expect that zinger that erases anything positive that has been said. They shut down, and the impact of the information you provide will be missed.

For this reason, it can be a good idea to separate the Positive Feedback you provide from this Formative Coaching. Instead, provide the majority of your Positive Feedback as close to the occurrence of the desired behavior as possible, and provide Formative Feedback at a time and in a place designated for review.

Hopefully, more often than not, the Formative Coaching you provide will involve the acknowledgment and reinforcement of successes. Setbacks, however, will occur, and should be addressed in a similarly routine manner. Don't jump in and take over, but model appropriate problem-solving behaviors. Discuss what happened using the step process/questions above.

Returning to our case study with Chad: his success was dependent on not only Positive and Descriptive Feedback – he needed to be taught, cajoled, and sometimes even pushed to see things differently. He needed to develop new skills, and to be taught how to use the skills he already possessed in a new and more fluid environment. This required the supportive feedback of Formative Coaching. And because of Chad's often rigid combative response when challenged to see or do things differently, much attention was paid to its delivery and timing.

These were tough conversations, but they always began with an honest discussion of where Chad stood. First, a review of all of his hard work, his determination and focused effort. And then, and only then, a review of his current difficulties, and the absolute and urgent need for improvement, for change.

With time, Chad came to understand that those providing feedback were in fact ***on his side***, and focused on helping him achieve his goal. He wanted an increased level of coaching, but also needed it to be predictable and consistent. For that reason, the preparatory and the post-evaluation coaching questions were used in scheduled reviews at the beginning and end of each day. ***It became routine, standard, and thus non-threatening.***

As a result, Chad was more open to whatever feedback he received, and he was much easier to work with - a win-win, you might say.

Final Thoughts

As you begin this transition, the quality of feedback you provide will be pivotal to the amount of growth your Breakaway can attain. Learn these different types of feedback, each with their own unique application, and utilize them as the key tools in your collaboration. Never forget timing, intention, and balance are all critical factors, and that a structured format will provide a "safe" atmosphere for criticism. Work to facilitate a culture where feedback can be provided and received with respect and trust.

Final Thoughts

- The quality of feedback you provide will be pivotal
- Learn the different types of feedback, each with their own unique application, and utilize them as key tools in your collaboration
- Never forget timing, intention, and balance are all critical factors
- A structured format will provide a "safe" atmosphere for criticism
- Work to facilitate a culture where feedback can be provided and received with respect and trust

Final Questions

1. Is there a specific type of feedback that you primarily find yourself using?
2. What type of feedback to you observe your spouse/partner primarily using?
3. Think of a time when the feedback you provided was well received and when it was not well received. What contributed to the outcome of each situation?
4. What in this chapter did you already know and feel comfortable implementing?
5. What in this chapter did you find most challenging, and possibly, most difficult to implement?
6. How do you think your Breakaway will respond to, your more intentional and strategic,

Notes

Commitment

One cannot be prepared for something while secretly believing it will not happen.

Nelson Mandela

The Breakaway

In 1519, Spanish conquistador Hernando Cortez, five thousand miles from home, on the shores of the Yucatan, and with no plan for reinforcement or resupply, ordered his men to "burn the ships". By doing so, he made a bold and uncompromising commitment to the challenge he and his men faced. And made history in the process.

Of course, the goal of that little expedition was to seize the treasure of the Aztec empire, but putting greed and colonization aside, Cortez's instincts as a leader were exactly right. All too aware they were greatly outnumbered in a distant land, he knew neither success nor their survival was guaranteed. With this decision, however, it would be all or nothing. He could not allow any of his roughly 600 men to waver in their dedication for a moment once hardship set in. Cortez needed them steely-eyed, hungry, focused on problem-solving their way forward, rather than looking for a means to avoid or retreat.

Their only option now was "Forward!"

As you can imagine, these orders were met with some resistance. In fact, he risked all-out mutiny. But his steadfast determination was infectious. The ships were burned. Cortez had just inspired the commitment of others, and instilled in them a belief they could rise to meet any future obstacles. It was this investment and faith that ensured their eventual victory – where others, over six centuries, had failed – in conquering the vast empire (sorry, Aztecs).

That is leadership.

And, in all likelihood, that is the level of commitment it will take for you and your developing young adult to navigate this period of change.

While it will (hopefully) not be necessary to burn ships, your home or car, it is incumbent upon you as leader to set the tone for this expedition.

Of all the elements discussed in this book, commitment is simultaneously the most important and also the most difficult to master. For unlike the rest, it begins and ends in one's heart. It is a sincere belief in the direction one has chosen and rock-solid determination to follow through. This requires genuine self-reflection and a willingness to face one's own doubts and fears. There is no shortcut. It cannot be faked.

But once felt, and declared, it is highly contagious...

It can excite and inspire the Breakaway into taking bold steps and accomplishing goals greater than they ever imagined.

Moving Forward (Only)

Moving forward means just that.

Your young adult cannot expect to maintain forward momentum with one foot in the comfort of home and high school and one foot in the newness and challenge of young adulthood. It won't work. This same principle applies to you. It is not possible to be an effective leader during this transition if one is not committed to a strategy of moving forward – *if one has secretly-held beliefs that it should or will not happen.*

It involves the construction of a new and clearly articulated reality, one where a retreat back to the relative safety of home, high school, and earlier stages of development, is just not possible. This is where many parents become paralyzed. Anxieties run high, and there is often great fear to make any move at all, for a fear that all progress made to this point will be lost.

As tough as it might seem, however, every great journey must start with that clear line of demarcation of before and after. If your goal is a life of greater independence for your son or daughter, you need to set a tone that clearly sends the message there is no going back. What this independence ultimately looks like is not the point. That will take shape as you gain momentum and things unfold. Let go of the idea it is possible to control everything and the need to have guarantees. Neither is possible. Instead, set a tone that expects, and appropriately pushes for, evolution and advancement rather than more of the same. Fully commit yourself to problem-solving your way through the adversity that is sure to come.

Your Breakaway may show signs of eager anticipation for the adventure ahead, and for the whole idea of change, only to be caught off guard when they fully realize the sheer number of challenges to be faced. *It is then they will quickly lose excitement for moving forward, as well as faith in their abilities. It is then they will need a strong leader.*

A leader that has a sturdy, stubborn plan based in reality, and unfaltering commitment to stay the course - despite their (and your own) very real nerves.

Of course, as no one's personal history, life experiences or presenting deficits are the same, the timing and process of establishing this line of demarcation will vary.

Below are a few examples that illustrate the experience of families with whom I have worked. The chronology of their stories may differ, but the ultimate outcomes are the same. They were all able to establish that Point Of No Return, where forward was the only logical option; where there was no need to look back and no impulse to retreat.

Bonnie

Bonnie's parents began to build their own commitment to this transition when she was only in ninth grade. They started planning for life after high school even as it was just beginning, primarily because Bonnie was slow to integrate new ideas into her way of thinking. They wanted to introduce the idea of independence early and often, with the hope she would become forward-thinking. They wanted her to develop the skill of looking beyond daily struggles toward broader goals.

They also very much wanted to be an example to Bonnie, by being forward-thinking and solution-focused themselves.

While this might seem like a difficult task to take on without eliciting fear and anxiety, their first step did not involve anything complicated. They simply started by stating their expectation, that just like her brother, Bonnie would achieve the highest level of independence her strengths and weaknesses would allow. And that this would involve living outside of Mom and Dad's home.

The details of how this would occur were not important. Instead, Bonnie's parents were focused on the establishment of an overall direction, a mindset of pushing forward.

The beauty of this approach was it gave Bonnie and her parents a lot of time – always a precious commodity – to get a clear assessment of her strengths and weaknesses. This enabled them to anticipate both areas of risk and opportunity, and to develop a plan for managing both. This time also enabled Bonnie's parents to contain their own anxiety about this transition, and bolster their own internal confidence to take it all on.

By the time of Bonnie's graduation, a well-conceived Strategic Plan was in place, and there was no doubt in anyone's minds Bonnie would build a life beyond her parents' home. Graduation then was a time for celebrating this great achievement, and a time of eager anticipation for Bonnie's next stage of development.

Jenna

In contrast to the approach taken with Bonnie, Jenna's parents had always been unsure about what she was capable of achieving. She had deficits in multiple areas, her social skills were much delayed, and approaches at skill-building were complicated by the difficult and tragic circumstances she confronted before her adoption. Friendships were limited or nonexistent, and had mostly been defined by teasing. As an only child, Jenna also missed the opportunity to build social skills within the more supportive environment of home and family. Together, these experiences magnified Jenna's insecurity, her feelings she was of no value and her general sense of rejection by the world. It also heightened her parents' anxieties, and their determination to cause no more harm.

Wanting to build her sense of self-esteem and to protect her from further rejection, Jenna's parents opted to home-school. In this environment they knew they could surround her with the love and support she needed to grow up healthy and happy. They wanted to be sure Jenna avoided further rejection. In this they were successful.

That is, until Jenna turned twenty-one, and it no longer seemed appropriate for her to have such a limited life experience. Jenna's parents had also tired of their role as sole caregivers, companions, best friends, coach, etc. They had become increasingly interested in the freedom they would experience by having Jenna live on her own.

To no one's surprise, Jenna was not excited about the idea when it was first presented. She was comfortable, and could see no logical reason why she should step away from the support, ease, and luxury that she enjoyed. Her parents, however, had found a new resolve, and were determined to facilitate this transition into greater independence. Jenna needed to become more independent, and they were going to make this happen.

Their first step involved enrolling Jenna in a local, residential-based program. While she could still come for visits, Jenna would not be living at home. She would be developing her new skill-set in a real world environment. This turned out to be a great move. While challenging for all involved, Jenna experienced much growth, and was increasingly confident with her new-found independence.

After a year in this program however, Jenna's focus continued to be on her return home, and on her desire not to grow up. She was compliant in her approach to this new set of expectations, but she had never really bought into the final goal. Being an adult was too scary, and included challenges she would rather avoid. Jenna preferred having others make the tough decisions about money, and food, and friends, and jobs.

Wanting to re-establish forward momentum, Jenna's parents made the tough decision to cut off her escape route. Despite their fear Jenna would experience any new effort to push her toward independence as rejection, they decided to establish a clear line of demarcation.

They told Jenna that just like her peers, it was time to become a young adult. It was time to establish herself in her own apartment. Time to be separate from Mom and Dad. They told Jenna she would always be welcome home, but her stays would more accurately be defined as visits. Their home was no longer her primary residence.

Finally, they told Jenna that her former bedroom was being converted into a combination office/guest room. The walls would no longer be pink, and her Pocahontas bedspread would be changed to something more neutral.

It was done. They had "burned the ships". They had clearly established Jenna's point of demarcation. There was no going back to childhood. Forward was now Jenna's only option. And forward she went. Jenna began to change. She began to identify with more mature peers, the challenges they were overcoming, their efforts to find employment. With time, she became more focused on her own skill development, and came to embrace the many opportunities that adulthood and independence would bring. She no longer looked to avoid growing up. She was looking forward. She was becoming a young adult.

Jenna now lives independently in an apartment with limited support, and has maintained part-time employment with the assistance of a job coach. Her parents are overjoyed with her progress, and Jenna is quite pleased with the level of independence she has achieved.

Dustin

The case example of Dustin falls somewhere in-between the previous two examples, as expectations for greater independence were not established until late into his senior year. Getting through the challenges of high school had always been his parents' primary focus. So it was not until an IEP meeting in Dustin's senior year when questions of transition shocked everyone into action. From that point forward, their collective focus and determination shifted to this next stage of development.

It was then that everything changed. Dustin's parents enlisted the support of a psychologist and transition team, with a renewed focus on having Dustin take responsibility for those daily chores and responsibilities he would need to make routine before going out on his own. Dustin's parents stopped doing his homework assignments, and they made a calculated decision to let Dustin struggle.

Just like his sisters, Dustin was told he could not live at home forever, and that at some point he would be expected to generate his own source of income. Support would be provided to assure he obtained the education and training he needed, but establishing himself as an independent young man was the ultimate goal.

They reminded Dustin their hope and expectation for his future was for him to find happiness, success and independence. They also reminded him he already possessed the skills to make this possible. If he was ever to get in the driver's seat of his own life, he needed to nurture and practice these skills under their supervision

With limited resistance, Dustin embraced this challenge, and those he faced after graduation. He learned to face adversity by first trying to find his own solutions before asking for assistance. He developed a good understanding for how his deficits affected him in school and on a daily basis, and how to advocate for support.

He learned to function independently and is doing well. Dustin is currently working very hard to complete his Bachelor's Degree in Geography.

Finding your Own Resolve

Whether you have been discussing this transition for several years or several months, now is the time to commit. Begin with reading back through the journal you have been creating while reading this book; a personal testament that highlights and helps you fully understand the uniqueness of your own situation. Look at problems and possible solutions with fresh eyes. Step away from any approach based in fear, the avoidance of all that could go wrong. Better to reach out towards the many positive possibilities, so your Breakaway embraces that outlook as well.

Obviously, it is not possible to protect your young adult from hardship, rejection, or the limitations they will face because of their deficits.

Nor should you want to!

It is my belief we are all obligated, as adults in their lives, to encourage (and teach) these Breakaways to increase their skills through a controlled process of meeting problems, rejecting a stance of victimhood, and facing the world with a determination to adapt and overcome. This is the resiliency needed to maximize their potential. Thus, we cannot overprotect out of concern for their welfare, or expect too much too soon out of a sense of urgency.

Finding this equilibrium is likely to feel near-impossible at times – trust me, I know – and will require an enormous amount of experimentation.

Remember: tailoring the size and shape of your support to fit the specific needs of the individual Breakaway is more important than any other factor when guiding this population.

Along with a willingness to truly commit, and to lead.

You and your aspiring young adult are facing a journey with an uncertain destination. This is simply the nature of transition.

It is also what makes the journey so exciting and worthwhile.

Forward!

Five Basic Principles to Bring with You on This Journey

1. **Understand the nature of your Breakaway's strengths and weaknesses.** The specific scaled scores on intelligence, academic achievement, psychological, neurological tests, yes – but beyond, on a more nuanced personal level. Understand their significance as they will affect the challenges of daily living for the recognizable future. Openly discuss this with them. Share ways you think they might work over, around or through weaknesses, and encourage them to do the same, to always be problem-solving. This prepares them for expecting and applying themselves in a more complex environment, to discover new skills and a higher level of confidence.

2. **Be strong!** Expect turbulence; recognize it as normal, and proactively ride it out. Encourage the exploration of skills and abilities in the world and do not expect perfection. Encourage fun in learning, and allow your young adult to experience some discomfort. It promotes skill development when combined with appropriate levels of structure and coaching. Resist the temptation to rush in and fix your young adult's struggles. Unexpected delays and surprises are part of the journey. Parachuting in robs them of the chance to develop the resilience that all adults need.

3. **Be consistent and set expectations.** Be consistent with your message of support and with your follow-through of limits and rules. We all thrive on clear expectations. If you are not demanding some level of self-sufficiency as a goal, your young adult will not strive to reach it. Remember, it is always better to build than to tear down. The privilege of independence must be earned. Set benchmarks for demonstrated success, rewarding skill development with greater freedom and responsibility. This approach recognizes the challenges they face and acknowledges developmental gains when they occur. The consequence of providing too much freedom and responsibility too soon are higher levels of anxiety, and damaging feelings of failure when previously granted freedoms are removed to fit the individual's skill level.

4. **Be patient.** Each young adult is on their own unique journey. Expect delays. Avoid the trap of prematurely expecting your young adult to navigate a less-structured environment without support.

5. **Seek out support and guidance.** Nothing about this transition into young adulthood is easy. The outside perspective of a psychologist knowledgeable of this population and this transition will be invaluable.

Notes

Notes

Appendix

Parent Notes & Extended Case Study

The Breakaway

The information contained in this appendix is a representative sample of a journal and plan, developed by the parents of a Breakaway facing this big transition - **Bryce**. This document is a compilation of all relevant and available information at the time of its creation. It includes all known challenges, opportunities, and potential traps Bryce and his family anticipated as he faced the transition to college or work, life outside his parent's home and greater independence. It also shows how they worked to develop long-term goals and a step-by-step plan for achieving them. Together, I believe these documents represent a great example of an approach you might take.

To provide context, I have included some information on Bryce below.

Bryce

Bryce was planning to move out of his parent's home for the upcoming Spring semester at a local Community College. He presented with a history of difficulties related to general developmental delays, poor social perception, limited emotional resilience, and executive functioning difficulties. He had received much assistance and special education services from an early age, relying completely on his parents to stay organized and to generally function on a daily basis.

Bryce's primary diagnosis was Autistic Spectrum Disorder (ASD). Cognitive and Academic testing classified him as 2e, and he had secondary diagnoses of Major Depression – Moderate, and Attention Deficit Hyperactivity Disorder – Combined Type. Additionally Bryce struggled with sensory integration issues and had both fine and gross coordination difficulties.

Bryce struggled to relate with others, to work on tasks requiring flexibility of thought, and had a restricted range of interests. He also struggled to organize himself, his thoughts and environment, and was a very slow processor of information.

Bryce's strengths were found in his demonstrated ability to work very hard, and in his great desire to be successful in everything he attempted. This determination had paid off, and he was now being given the opportunity to live on his own and go to college, where the support he needed could no longer be provided by his parents.

Despite his previous success, everyone involved was well aware this next step was going to be challenging. He was good in familiar situations, but would backslide with newness. When faced with unpracticed tasks or ones requiring the rapid processing of information, organizational skills or flexibility, Bryce's work slowed significantly. At times he might even avoid these tasks entirely. New situations, even when requiring the use of well-practiced skills, were sometimes just too much for him to handle on his own. The overwhelming nature of the challenge his deficits presented also made it enormously difficult for Bryce to develop new skills.

None of these challenges, however, were viewed as a reason for Bryce to avoid this next step toward greater independence. The resulting anxiety experienced by his parents was actually a motivator. Instead of sticking to the relative safety of what they had known to work, they started to develop a plan. One that made sense for Bryce and everyone providing support.

This process started when Bryce's parents and psychologist sat down and discussed the situation. Together, they began to develop a plan based on a thorough evaluation of his strengths and weaknesses, and the advances and skills required for Bryce to reach his goals.

This is what they created. Consider how you might do the same:

Notes – Page 1

Strengths Observed in Bryce & Parents

- Bryce is good in situations once he has become familiar.
- Bryce has strong verbal skills.
- Bryce is attractive and can be charming.
- Well liked by adults in his life. – Teachers, counselors, etc.
- Bryce wants to grow up and become independent.
- Parents are able to financially support Bryce through this transition.
- Bryce has the cognitive ability to manage college if he is willing/able to work through his deficits, accept accommodations, and focus on developing his own work-arounds.
- Everyone in the family is still working to understand how Bryce's deficits will impact him in the "real world" – and are okay with this ambivalence.
- Bryce is very determined and has expressed a strong desire to continue school.
- Parents also report significant desire to step away from the day to day concerns of Bryce's behavior and emotions.
- Counseling will be available for emotional support and encouragement, and as a rational voice to normalize typical stressors. For both Bryce and parents.
- Parents willing to let Bryce struggle in the process of learning, as long as external supports are in place. Psychologist to help with this.
- Responds well to routines.
    - We will plug in apartment checks and skill development sessions three times per week.
    - Bryce will also be given a weekly schedule to follow.
- Parents express desire not to be "helicopter parents" but acknowledge that this will be very hard.
    - Still conflicted over idea of Bryce moving out of family home. Many associated fears.
    - Parents open to outside support, and are putting this in place.

Notes – Page 2

Weaknesses Observed in Bryce and Parents

- Bryce presents with deficits in the processing of information, that is often further impaired, by newness and stress.
- Bryce is at times unrealistic about what he is capable of achieving.
- We have some fear that Bryce's determination to achieve independence will limit his willingness to ask for, or accept, help when he needs it.
- Mom's role with Bryce has been that of advocate and fixer during tough times. We anticipate that Bryce will struggle to take on the responsibility of these roles in the early phases of this transition.
- Parents are struggling to get Bryce to practice the skills he will need to have mastered (laundry, cooking, shopping, using alarm clock, getting up without reminders, wearing a watch, etc.) prior to moving out on his own.
- In most areas of needed growth, Bryce appears to be in stage two within the Change Model. Areas of great interest to him however, fit better in stage three.
- Limited experience managing meds with complete independence.
    - Need to develop a system for monitoring.
    - At this point Bryce reports desire to remain med compliant.
- Bryce is likely to have difficulty applying information learned in one situation or interaction to others.
    - Ongoing coaching will be important. Who? How often?
    - Build into role of counselor and daily support providers.
- Bryce has deficits in the organization of information, his thoughts, himself, his choices, and his environment. These weaknesses are very prominent when stressed, tired, or when in new environments.
- Bryce has in large part, depended on others to identify goals and to set a direction for achievement.
    - Must help him take this role on for himself.
    - Money mgmt., getting up on time, and managing his apartment should be areas of focus.
- Bryce struggles with the pragmatics of social interaction, often resulting in poor communication and poor peer relationships.
    - Psychologist will continue to address.
    - Will introduce him to peer group for students with similar challenges with hopes that he may build some friendships.
- Bryce is determined, but struggles to focus on more than one thing at a time. His resilience will be limited as resource depletion will be significant.

Notes - Page 3

Weaknesses Observed in Bryce and Parents - Cont.

- History of depression that may affect his resiliency.
- Struggles to understand others when their perceptions are different from his own.
- Limited flexibility of thought - especially when stressed.
- Avoids the unfamiliar.
- Backslides when confronted with new situations.
- Fine and gross motor coordination skill deficits.
- Poor organizational skills/executive functioning.

Threats To Forward Momentum

- Emotional instability related to his history of depression.
- His natural identity development process may result in an evolution of more rebellious and noncompliant behavior as he matures. Developmentally Bryce feels twelve or thirteen in most areas. Will need to navigate this with him, as his he matures.
- We are concerned that Bryce may decide not to take his meds as a way of proving he is "just like everyone else".
- Bryce's ideas of what college and life after high school is like, are largely based on images he has seen in the movies and tv. Not sure how he will respond to the realities of studying, stress, and increased expectations for responsibility.
- If he is stressed and chooses not to do this anymore, we are not sure how we would respond. We are not excited about him living with us forever.
- We have limited financial realities. If job statuses change, or if Bryce needs loads of long-term support, our current level of support will have to be reduced.
- Poor choices with peers, or decisions to experiment with drugs and alcohol could upend our progress.
- Mom in more reluctant than dad to push Bryce, and to let him experience failure.
  - Bryce sometimes uses this difference to manipulate.
- Bryce has a history of multiple failures and the desire to avoid a continuation of this experience.

  - What will this mean when he faces the predictable and normal setbacks/adversity of college and independence?

Notes – Page 4

Opportunities During This Transition

- The support team we have found presents an opportunity for Bryce to see what he can do for himself in a world of greater independence.
- Moving out of mom and dad's house will let me be like friends in high school.
- This is a great time to see what I can do in the world on my own.
- The availability of a program that will let me learn to live independently, and help me with college.
- With Bryce out of the home, we can finally take a vacation.
- There is a film school within the local college system.
- With the other students in the program I should be able to make friends.
- Maybe I could ask friends over for dinner, or to play video games.
- Maybe I will get a girlfriend.
- Changing environments from home to an apartment will provide a great opportunity to mature.
- Bryce is at times unrealistic about what he is capable of achieving.

Notes - Page 5

"Unspoken" Parental Concerns About The Plan

- Bryce will experience a reasonably high level of stress, as this transition will require the acquisition of new skills, and the confrontation of old fears and anxieties.

- How will Bryce's deficits impact his ability to navigate, and to advocate for himself within a college bureaucracy?

- Freshman housing is typically in a dorm with a roommate. Will need to see if a single dorm room, or off campus apartment is possible.

- We believe that Bryce is more scared than he is letting on.

- We are afraid that Bryce will not be successful in his attempts to live independently, and to be self-sufficient.

- What if he can't find friends?

- Bryce expressed no concern/fear about this transition. He is primarily focused on the idea of independence. Does he know what that means?

- Given his history of depress who will monitor his mood?

- We are concerned that we will not be able to communicate with professors, administrators, and the university in general.

  –Who will help him with this?
  –Is there someone in the Student Access Center that will get him.

  Can Bryce navigate this with his executive functioning deficits?
  ** Review with support team.

- While we have money set aside for college, available funds are limited. Bryce must make progress in a reasonable timeframe, or a shift to a job/vocational track will be considered.

- What if the support team we have in place cannot help us?

Notes - Page 6

Themes that Define Bryce's Approach to Things

- I can do just as much as anyone else!
- Slow & steady
- Anything but the label of disability
- At times - Crisis and overwhelmed
- What if I can't do it

Themes that Define Mom's Approach to Things

- Get it done!
- Don't tell us it can't be done
- Anxiety fueled OCD

Themes that Define Dad's Approach to Things

- Slow & Steady
- Generally calm and methodical
- Everything works its self out with time and patience
- Focus

Notes – Page 7

Info on Cognitive & Academic Current Functioning

WISC-V

	IQ Score	Range	Percentile
Verbal Comprehension	133	Extremely High	99th
Visual Spatial	95	Average	45th
Fluid Reasoning	110	Average	74th
Working Memory	86	Low Average	17th
Processing Speed	83	Low Average	13th
General Ability Index	115	High Average	16th
Cognitive Proficiency Index	91	Average	30th

Woodcock-Johnson Test of Achievement

	Standard Score	Percentile Band	Grade Equivalent
Brief Achievement	99	96-101	11.6
Broad Math	85	82-88	9
Basic Reading Skills	100	97-104	12
Brief Math	90	86-93	9.4
Math Calculations	79	75-84	8.6
Basic Writing Skills	105	101-109	12.2
Academic Skills	96	94-99	10.9
Academic Fluency	85	95-101	11.1
Phon/Graph Know	98	95-100	11.1
Letter-Word Identification	102	98-106	12.2
Reading Fluency	94	90-98	10.2
Calculation	85	80-91	9.1
Math Fluency	75	72-78	1.8
Spelling	101	96-106	12
Writing Fluency	89	83-95	9.1
Applied Problems	95	91-98	9.6
Word Attack	99	96-103	11
Editing	107	103-111	12
Spelling of Sounds	94	89-99	9.1

Need to understand what these skills mean for Bryce on a daily basis!

Notes - Page 8
Categories for Existing Abilities

Knowing, Doing, & Maintaining

- Sets alarm and gets out of bed on-time
- General hygiene skills - tooth brushing not always
- Positive social behaviors - hand shaking, introductions, eye contact etc.
- When given a schedule he will follow

Knowing, Doing with Prompts and Support

- Brushing teeth
- Advocating for his needs or accommodations setting other than home
- Academic/study skills - has had the structure of tutors and support
- Money management - has not managed more than allowance
- Cleaning room or putting dishes in dishwasher
- Needs prompts to get haircuts
- Organizational skills
- Emotional self-regulation
- Struggles to modulate the volume of voice

Knowing, Learning to do with Much Support

- Laundry
- Managing and creating own daily schedule
- Continues to need support in creating and maintaining friendships
- Completing forms in school or medical settings - forgets address, SS#, and phone numbers without a key.

Limited Knowledge and Doing Skills

- Meal prep and grocery shopping - other than cereal
- Public transportation - not a driver
- Never has lived independently or been away from home for extended period of time
- Has not yet had a job

Notes - Page 9
Specific Areas of Strength & Weakness To Consider

Executive Functioning

- Bryce's executive functioning abilities are limited. He struggles to manage his behavior and to cope with his emotions generally.
- Bryce has deficits in the organization of information, his thoughts, himself, his choices, and his environment. These weaknesses are very prominent when stressed, tired, or when in new environments.

Sensory Processing

- Bryce is often bothered by the texture of foods. He does not like to stand too close to others and thinks he always notices when someone lightly touches his arm or back. Bryce can also be sensitive to loud noises - especially when tired and stressed.

Other Observations

- Bryce presents with deficits in the processing of information, that is often further impaired by newness and stress.
- Bruce is at times unrealistic about what he is capable of achieving.
- We have some fear that Bryce's determination to achieve independence will limit his willingness to ask for, or accept help when he needs it.
- Bryce can make friends but struggles to know what to do to maintain friendships.
- Bryce is determined
- He generally is a rule follower
- He reports no concern about graduating high school
- He is at times immature

History of Accommodations

- Extended time to complete all tests
- Has received remedial math instruction
- He needs extra support and instruction on how to organize school materials
- Teachers and tutors should check in on his progress regularly to be sure that he is both on task and making good progress with his work.
- He struggles to identify the demands of some tasks. He thus will need instruction in how to assess a given task and approach it in a methodical was. This is especially true in math.
- He benefits from quick-reference notes from the instructor. These help him to identify key information, and rules and strategies that apply to any given type of math problem.

Notes – Page 10

Specific Areas of Strength & Weakness To Consider

Skills of Independence

- Bryce is able to shower, bath, brush teeth etc., but is known to not complete these tasks without prompting.
- Bryce does not drive. He has some, but minimal, experience with public transportation.
- Bryce's skills for money management are limited. He struggles to track his spending.
- Bryce does not yet do his own laundry.
- Bryce is not currently able to prepare his own meals or grocery shop with independence. He has some experience with both.
- Bryce struggles to maintain a clean organized bedroom.
- Bryce is compliant with taking his meds when we sit them out in the morning. Not sure if he could do this without prompting.
- Bryce can tell-time, but requires prompting to follow his schedule. The is true outside of school when bells are not available to signal transitions.
- Bryce communicates well with others – especially when he needs something.
- Bryce has not managed medical appointments on his own.

Strengths

- Hard worker
- Desire to be successful

Weaknesses

- Bryce is slow to adjust to change – although when he has a routine and understands expectations his functioning increases greatly.
- Slow processor of information
- At times struggles to manage his energy and emotions.

Diagnoses

Autism Spectrum Disorder
ADHD
Depression
Sensory Integration Disorder

Notes – Page II

Open Questions

- How will Bryce be limited by his low math skills and processing speed? Will this limit his academic and vocational opportunities?
- Will Bryce's skills for self-regulation improve with age?
- Do we need to update his testing if he is to receive accommodations going forward?
- What accommodations will be most appropriate?
- Will Bryce be able to have a roommate or should he live alone?
- Is living at home for a year a better option?
- Who other than us can provide support going forward?
- What do we need to do now to prepare Bryce?
- Will he be able to step-up to the challenge?
- Can we afford to get Bryce the support he needs?
- Are Voc Rehab or SSI a resource that Bryce qualifies for?
- What do we need to put in place to support him in the long term?

After a review of the notes, generated over time and many conversations, Bryce's parents developed their own Strategic Mission and plan of action. By putting this in writing they felt these efforts going forward would be more focused and unified. This became their guide for the direction taken, and to inform individual goal setting. These are:

Notes – Page 12

Parental Strategic Mission: Goal Setting & Next Steps

- Efforts to support Bryce will not be designed to alter the expectations that he will face in the world with his academics or work, but rather, will focus on teaching him the skills to work around his unique obstacles, and to facilitate the use of accommodations when appropriate.

- In order to foster an environment of growth and development, Bryce will be given the opportunity to "graduate" to higher levels of independence as he demonstrates success and readiness for all that entails. it is hoped that this approach will foster a culture where he will more readily seek out support in an effort to gain the skills needed to become independent – and where there are identifiable reasons for him to confront his anxiety to learn new things.

- A culture of punishment and limit setting should be avoided. We want to build from success, more than we want to take away responsibilities that were prematurely granted.

- Bryce will be expected to follow a higher level of structure for at least one semester to provided an opportunity to demonstrate skill development in the areas of time mgmt., self-regulation, and the mgmt. of his emotions.

- We want Bryce to demonstrate the ability to make appointments, sustain a consistent effort, and to stay reasonably organized, before expecting him to take on the responsibilities of greater independence – and thus lower levels of supervision and structure.

    –Attendance to class/tutoring/study hall, counseling appointments, and self mgmt. within apartment will be used as basic measures of these skills.

- Bryce will be asked to bring fewer numbers of personal and luxury items (gaming systems) with him to his apartment until he has demonstrated the ability to manage the basics – and most importantly to develop healthy routines. Routines cannot occur when overwhelmed by one's personal environment.

Establishing a Strategic Direction - Setting Goals

Their next step was to sit with Bryce to identify some long-term goals and the skills he would need to reach them. They wanted him to be fully engaged, to have a greater awareness of what was ahead, and most especially, they wanted his feedback and buy-in.

Notes – Page 13

Long-Term Goals for Bryce

- Bryce will develop the skills necessary to live independently with success.
- Bryce will develop the means to, at least in part, financially support himself.
- Bryce will learn to manage his emotions sufficiently to face the challenges of each day.
- Bryce will go to class even if feeling anxious or scared.
- Bryce will go to class even if feeling anxious or scared.
- Bryce will independently advocate for the assistance and accommodations he needs at school and work.
- Bryce will develop a network of friends.
- Bruce will feel okay with his deficits.
- Bryce will earn a college degree.
- Bryce will learn to distinguish typical daily stressors, from an emotional crisis.
- Bryce will take his medication as prescribed.
- Bryce will create a happy life for himself.
- Bryce will maintain a safe and healthy apartment.
- Bryce will maintain a healthy diet.
- Bryce will find a career field that fits his specific skill set.
- Bryce will develop the skills needed to maintain full-time employment.
- Bryce will maintain his own daily schedule within a day planner or Smart Phone calendar program.
- Bryce will go to film school.
- Bryce will become a professional movie director.

Once they completed their list of potential goals, and Bryce was on-board, the family was asked to identify those foundational skills needed (those Bryce did not already possess) to achieve all, or even a small group of, these goals. The skill gaps identified would guide the development of Short-Term Objectives and Action Plans for achievement. To their credit, the family was able to quickly come to an agreement on eight areas of weakness, in need of significant refinement. These areas were:

Notes – Page 14

Skills needed To Reach Goals

- *Bryce's ability to plan ahead*
- *The ability to stay organized without assistance*
- *Bryce's ability to manage stress*
- *Bryce's awareness of time*
- *Bryce needs to take his meds without mom's prompting*
- *Bryce's ability to match his emotions to the situation in which he finds himself*
- *Bryce's ability to shower daily and brush teeth without prompting*
- *Interpersonal and social skills appropriate to his age, and situation*

Next Steps

Given that Bryce and his family had decided to enroll him in a support program for the upcoming semester, many of the details associated with working toward these goals were already in place. While this was a nice surprise, it did not mean however the family would be skipping the very important step of engaging Bryce in the development of specific short-term objectives. He and his parents clearly identified, and agreed upon, the specific steps Bryce needed to take in order to achieve his goals. Handing things off to the support program was never considered. Doing this would have resulted in the disengagement of everyone involved, and would not have modeled the self-efficacy and responsibility that everyone wanted Bryce to develop.

In my experience, failure to pause and go through the steps of self assessment and Action Planning results in confusion, and a tendency for parents to unnecessarily intervene for their Breakaway. Teachable moments are then lost as they have no need to find their own solutions. Within a support program setting, this disconnect can also result in a misperception that "the program" is imposing arbitrary and uncomfortable expectations, again "necessitating" parental intervention.

As a general rule, all unnecessary, disruptive, and unhelpful activity results from the absence of a unifying plan among those providing support. Without a unifying and consistent conceptual plan, it becomes impossible to know when to provide assistance and when to let a situation play itself out. Interventions become random and inconsistency becomes the rule.

The program they found was outstanding, but it still required them to be engaged in the change that was about to unfold.

With support from the entire team, Bryce and his family then developed Short-Term Objectives that were categorized into three specific areas: *Executive Functioning, Emotional Functioning,* and *Social Functioning*. This was done so that the scope of all conversations going forward would focus not only on the specific behavior, but also the general area of functioning in which each skill or behavior is based.

Doing this made it easier to ask those questions that got to the root of any specific area of struggle, and to appropriate strategies for providing support.

On the next page are the Short-Term Objectives that were developed.

Notes – Page 15

Short-Term Objectives

Executive Functioning

- Bryce will independently manage his medication
- Bryce's spending on food and recreation will stay within his established budget
- Bryce will attend all of his scheduled appointments at the appropriate time and location

Social

- Bryce will develop a small group of friends
- Bryce will maintain age appropriate hygiene by showering daily, and by brushing his teeth once in the morning, and once at bedtime.

  **This could have been listed under executive functioning, but was more motivating for Bryce when approached from a social angle.

Emotional

- Bruce will express his feelings of anger, frustration and anxiety in an age appropriate manner, by using his words and writing in his journal.
- Bryce will meet with his counselor once weekly.

The Structure Behind Skill Building

Now that short-term objectives were identified in three key areas of need, it was time to get down to the specifics, of building skills. The first step for Bryce started with making decisions about the level and type of external support he required. Since Bryce had no previous experience living on his own, he needed guidance and support so that the challenges he faced were congruent with his ability to manage them, and to grow through the experience. It was decided he would respond best to an approach that validated the anxiety, fear and ambivalence he was experiencing, while at the same time presenting opportunities for him to explore the consequences of his choices.

Bryce was being given more freedom to choose than he had ever had before, but was also being provided with a support system to keep him headed in the right direction: one with checks-and-balances designed to teach, hold him accountable, and to monitor his ability to manage this responsibility. Rather than expecting he take full responsibility for developing and managing his own schedule, Bryce was provided with a weekly schedule to follow. This took away the need for him to make decisions about what to do, where to go, and when to be there. However, it kept in place the responsibility of time management, navigation from one place to another, the need to keep track of his schedule, to call if he was going to be late or miss an appointment, and to fight his impulse to avoid when feeling anxious or depressed. It also provided plenty of opportunity to make mistakes. The structure provided for Bryce was designed to mirror and teach those executive functioning skills used by the most successful students and employees. Specifically, the efficient use of daylight hours to plan, to organize, and to complete one's work. This was a model he could take with him into adulthood.

Like many young college students, Bryce had not learned the art of studying during the day. He was more focused on doing his work in the evening, like he had done in high school. This however, would not be an effective model going forward because of increased demands and stressors. He needed time in the evening to recharge for the next day. With his limited executive functioning skills, it was also not realistic to expect Bryce to successfully complete work once he was back in his apartment.

He still required the support of tutors. He also needed to learn a routine for starting his day in the morning, putting forth a persistent effort until his work was complete, and getting to bed at a reasonable hour. He could no longer afford to stay up all night and sleep late the next day. Uncomfortable as these changes might be, these skills would last him a lifetime.

After a while, it was expected (hoped) he would internalize these routines, making them his own as he matured and became more able to define his own path.

To this end, whenever possible, Bryce was included in the process of developing his action plan.

The following is what they came up with.

Bryce's Approach to Executive Functioning Skill Development

While Bryce had previously been to classes designed to teach executive functioning skills, self-advocacy and goal setting, he had no opportunity to practice these skills outside of an artificial setting. As a result, very little of this information was absorbed or retained, and he struggled to transfer what he did retain to other settings, once faced with the fast-paced nature and expectations of daily living.

This is a familiar dilemma for anyone working to build skills with this population, so I am guessing it is consistent with your own experience. Individuals who struggle to sustain focus and attention, who struggle to process information efficiently, and who struggle to practically apply information learned in the abstract, tend not to retain information taught in a traditional classroom based or instructional format. ***Ironically, it takes executive functioning to learn executive functioning, only when all senses are engaged.*** As noted previously, Bryce needed the experiential learning that comes through operating in the real world. Below is a list of the initial Action Plans that Bryce himself developed:

Notes – Page 16

Executive Functioning – 1

Objective: Bryce will take his medication as prescribed.

Who: The responsibility for achieving this goal will be Bryce's. However, he will receive guidance and coaching through his support program to prevent significant lapses in this area.

What: Bryce's Meds are taken exclusively in the morning. A basic structure for the development of a routine will include:

1) The use of a monthly medication organizer.

2) Reminder alarms set on phone

3) Having Bryce send a text message each morning once he has taken his meds.

4) twice weekly checks by Bryce's support program to assure that the appropriate number of meds are missing from the med organizer – and to be sure that the appropriate alarms continue to be set on his phone.

When: Bryce will take his medication as prescribed with an 80% Success Rate.

While it was clearly important that Bryce's rate of Med. Compliance lie closer to 100%, Bryce and his team agreed that this was an acceptable first objective. Initial success and a reduced sense of pressure were important. Bryce expressed the complete intention to take his meds, but wanted to avoid perception of failure if he were not able to do this 100% of the time. This compliance rate was initially set at a level that could assure success.

Second only in difficulty to remembering to take his medication consistently, impulsive spending was the next big area of challenge for Bryce.

Notes – Page 17
Executive Functioning – 2

Objective: Bryce's spending for food and recreation will stay within his established budget.

Who: The responsibility for achieving this goal will be Bryce's. However, he will receive guidance and coaching through his support program to prevent significant lapses in this area.

What:
1) Bryce will meet once weekly with support staff to review his spending for the previous week, and to obtain money for the week ahead.

2) Bryce will first demonstrate his ability to manage his spending by first, only working with cash. This will provide both visual and tactile reminders of the money he is spending.

3) Bryce will be given total freedom to spend his recreational/ entertainment money as he chooses, but will not be given more once his budget money has been spent each week.

4) Bryce will initially be assisted with grocery shopping to assure that he buys the groceries he needs for each week.

When: Bryce will operate using this cash system for one semester, at which time a determination will be made about his readiness to manage the responsibility of his debut card. Opportunities to demonstrate this readiness will be provided as he graduates to managing both his recreation and food money without supervision, as he demonstrates the ability to have his money last the entire week, and as he demonstrates the ability to resist impulse spending.

The third area of executive Functioning to be addressed was the objective of being present and on-time to appointments. This was an area that had to improve if Bryce was to find success in college.

Notes – Page 18

Executive Functioning – 3

Objective: Bryce will attend all of his scheduled appointments at the appropriate time and location.

- This goal is seen as step-one toward Bryce's long-term goal of managing his own schedule. Our expectation is that, with time, Bryce will develop a high level of responsibility for his own schedule. For now however, following a schedule with greater independence is challenge one, toward this goal.

Who: It is Bryce's responsibility to follow his schedule, to have it with him at all times, and to ask for a new copy if it has been lost or misplaced.

What: 1) Before classes or tutoring begin, Bryce will receive support and coaching in finding the location of each of his appointments, and will practice navigating between them.

2) Bryce will be provided with a new paper copy of his schedule each week to account for possible changes in scheduled appointments. While minimal changes are expected, it is important that Bryce develop an awareness that changes to one's routine can occur, and that he learn to manage this reality.

3) Bryce will be assisted in setting alarms in his phone for each appointment, and with setting a morning alarm.

4) For one semester Bryce will receive a wake-up call in the morning to be sure that he is awake and moving.

5) The phone numbers of support staff will be programmed in Bryce's phone, so that he may call for assistance if feeling lost or confused.

6) Support staff will monitor Bryce's attendance to all appointments through direct observation, and by touting base with tutors, and other support staff.

When: Bryce will be present and on-time to 80% of his appointments each week for the semester.

149

Bryce's Approach to Improved Social Functioning

    The second key area of focus for Bryce was his ability to relate to others in a socially/age-appropriate manner. While not requiring organizational skills in the same way as cleaning one's apartment, the self-regulation required for social interaction is very clearly linked to executive functioning. And like all other areas of needed growth, the structure of the program made it easier for skill development as social opportunities were built into the experience, and his schedule.

    However, unlike the areas of executive and emotional functioning, instruction and coaching in the social arena was much more subtle and hands-off. This was one area where Bryce presented with a high level of internal motivation for change. He wanted a more mature, adult-to-adult relationship from his support providers. He just needed others to facilitate the development of his confidence, by gently guiding him through the choices he made about potential friends.

    As he gingerly navigated this new territory, the specifics of the action plans were in large part dictated by him. Still, in an effort to balance these dual needs of autonomy and support, social opportunities were "built in" to his weekly schedule. Typically there were four or five, either through his support program, or on-campus organizations. Bryce asked that his attendance be voluntary, and thus not subject to the same level of monitoring as other objectives.

    Below are the of action plans Bryce developed for this area of functioning.

Notes - Page 19

Social Functioning - 1

Objective: Bryce will develop a small group of friends.

Who: It is Bryce's responsibility to take advantage of available opportunities to meet and get to know his peers.

What: Weekly social opportunities either organized by his support program, or available on campus, will be included on Bryce's weekly schedule. These opportunities will be discussed with his adviser so that he is made aware of the specifics of each opportunity.

When: Bryce will attend one social opportunity each week. This may include an event organized on campus, through his support program, or informally with friends as these relationships develop.

During the process of developing action plans for this next objective, ("Bryce will maintain age appropriate hygiene by showering daily, and by brushing his teeth once in the morning, and once at bedtime"), Bryce and his parents came to realize that they combined two objectives into one. In order to facilitate effective feedback and reinforcement, this single objective was broken out into two distinct objectives.

Below are the two resulting Objectives and Action Plans:

Notes - Page 20

Social Functioning I-A

Objective I-A: Bryce will shower daily.

Who: Bryce is the responsible party for meeting this objective.

What: Bryce will be provided support in the form of four different tools or prompts. These are:

1) Reminder alarms set for the evening when Bryce has decided to shower.
2) Bryce will place a reminder note and an extra bottle of shampoo next to his alarm clock to serve as a prompt before he goes to bed.
3) Bryce will have a chart (including a pencil) taped to his bathroom mirror, for him to make a record of when he takes a shower.
4) Support staff will monitor Bryce's progress, being sure to focus on positive reinforcement and coaching as needed.

When: Bryce will shower 4 evenings per week.

Notes – Page 21
Social Functioning 1-B

Objective I-B: Bryce will brush his teeth twice daily. Once in the morning, and once in the evening.

Who: Bryce is the responsible party for meeting this objective.

What: Bryce will be provided support in the form of 5 different tools or prompts. These are:

1) Reminder alarms set to go off in the morning, and in the evening at a time chosen by Bryce.
2) Bryce will have a note over the toilet in his bathroom.
3) Bryce would like a toothbrush taped to the light switch in his bedroom to serve as a funny visual reminder.
4) Bryce will have a chart taped to his bathroom mirror, so that he may record when he brushes his teeth.
5) Support staff will monitor Bryce's progress being sure to focus on positive reinforcement and coaching as needed.

When: Bryce will brush his teeth eight times each week.

**This has been a particularly difficult task for Bryce to master. At present, Bryce's goal of brushing his teeth eight times per week is seen as a significant accomplishment. Expectations will be adjusted as Bryce demonstrates the consistent ability to meet this expectation.

Bryce's Approach to Improved Emotional Functioning

Bryce's emotional functioning, specifically his stress management skills, were another important area that impacted his overall functioning. Like everything else, they were linked to his capacity for self-regulation, and continued to be a significant area of difficulty. He was quick to catastrophize challenges faced, he struggled to know when and whom it was appropriate to express these emotions, and he struggled consistently to advocate for himself when in need of support.

Again, the external structure provided by his parents and support program was essential. Routine and stability in large areas of his life were essential. Within this relative stability he could experiment with and practice new or expanded coping skills.

Notes – Page 22

Emotional Functioning – 1

Objective: Bryce will express his feelings of anger, frustration and anxiety, in an age appropriate manner.

Who: Bryce is the responsible party for reaching this objective.

What:

1) Bryce will verbalize his feelings rather than physically taking them out on himself or others.

2) Bryce will continue to use his journal as a means of expressing his emotions.

3) Bryce will create a password protected document on his computer where he may journal his thoughts, feelings and experiences each day.

4) Bryce will have one hour each week of supportive counseling, where he may freely express his emotions and work through challenges of the week.

5) When present, support staff will positively reinforce Bryce's efforts to verbalize his thoughts and feelings, and will provide supportive coaching as needed.

When:

1) Bryce will attend his supportive counseling each week.
2) Bryce will journal 3 times weekly.

Notes – Page 23

Emotional Functioning – 2

Objective: Bryce will meet with his psychologist once weekly.

> ** Linked to the above objective, Bryce and his support team thought it important that his efforts to make this appointment were specifically acknowledged and reinforced.

Who: Bryce is the responsible party for developing and following through with this goal.

What:

1) Each week Bryce will receive a hard copy of his schedule that includes this appointment.

2) Reminder alarms will be placed on his phone.

3) When present, support staff will help focus Bryce's attention to his schedule by asking him; What he is currently doing?; What's next on his schedule?; and At what time he needs to be at his next appointment?

When: Bryce will be present and on-time to 80% of appointments with his psychologist.

With this structure in place, Bryce's plate was full.

Despite his occasional assertion to the contrary, Bryce very clearly needed support and direction. He was provided with a level of support and challenge appropriate to what was learned from their advanced planning and self-assessment. These efforts ultimately resulted in an intentional and well thought out approach to this transition that included checks and balances to prevent significant crashes while Bryce was learning to drive change, to make decisions, and to navigate adversity. Together they had successfully avoided the crisis mode of response that occurs with a lack of collaboration, planning, and understanding for the challenges to be faced.

His team, however, was also ready for surprises – prepared to provide more structure, or less, in response to his needs. Most importantly, Bryce had bought into the plan he and his team had developed for this transition. He was ready to go!

In my experience, the self-determination needed to take complete charge, only occurs once the developing young adult finds success in their own efforts, and when they are internally driven by a goal requiring these executive functioning skills.

Learning by doing is key here.

If you remain focused on learning, growth will occur. And learning comes only after a genuine Buy-In to the process, not just passive compliance.

If your developing young adult is unwilling or unable to engage in this process, it is perfectly acceptable to start with an intervention based in external structure, and expectations established by you and the world at large. Create dynamics where appropriate and natural consequences may occur, and avoid the impulse to jump in when they do occur. By all means be supportive, but allow this experiential learning to occur.

Notes

Notes

The Breakaway

Made in the USA
Columbia, SC
02 June 2023

17608092R00093